The Finch in My Brain

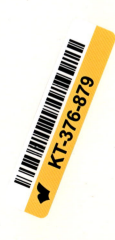
KT-376-879

The Finch in My Brain

Martino Sclavi

HODDER &
STOUGHTON

First published in Great Britain in 2017 by
Hodder & Stoughton
An Hachette UK company

1

Copyright © Martino Sclavi 2017

Chapter heading illustrations © Margarita Sclavi 2017, www.houseofita.com

The right of Martino Sclavi to be identified as the
Author of the Work has been asserted by him in accordance
with the Copyright, Designs and Patents Act 1988.

All rights reserved. No part of this publication may be reproduced,
stored in a retrieval system, or transmitted, in any form or by any means
without the prior written permission of the publisher, nor be otherwise
circulated in any form of binding or cover other than that in which it is published
and without a similar condition being imposed on the subsequent purchaser.

A CIP catalogue record for this title is available from the British Library

Hardback ISBN 978 1 473 64971 2
eBook ISBN 978 1 473 64973 6

Typeset in Simoncini Garamond Std and Optima by
Palimpsest Book Production Ltd, Falkirk, Stirlingshire

Printed and bound in Great Britain by Clays Ltd, St Ives plc

Hodder & Stoughton policy is to use papers that are natural,
renewable and recyclable products and made from wood grown in
sustainable forests. The logging and manufacturing processes are expected
to conform to the environmental regulations of the country of origin.

Hodder & Stoughton Ltd
Carmelite House
50 Victoria Embankment
London EC4Y 0DZ

www.hodder.co.uk

To all the nurses who put their emotions
at the forefront of their work

Contents

Chapters in Optima *are set before 2011, when Chapter One begins*

Foreword

It is eerily joyful to write a foreword to Martino Sclavi's book *The Finch in My Brain*, because five years ago I accepted that he was going to die. Not in a cosmic 'You gotta go sometime' way. No, I observed the face of the man in the white coat in the Kaiser Permanente Hospital as he held up a grim grey scan of Martino's brain. 'That dark area is the tumour,' he said. It was big. I mean, Tino has a big brain, as you'll discover when you read his book, but this malignant shadow, this dark fist, pushed the hemispheric boundary that runs through the brain into a dreadful bend.

'Is he going to be all right?' I asked.

That's when the man in the white coat did the face. He pulled his lips tight, his face tensed, his eyes were soft and certain and he tilted his head in a manner that brought the unbounded, rolling, taken-for-granted friendship of Martino into a sharp, tearful pinnacle. This was a face that they surely don't teach in Med School, but must be learned by the frequent conveyance of morbid news.

That night five years ago was as dark and grey as the scan. Sudden mortifying gluts that stained my mind as indelibly as the darkness that grew inside Martino's.

And yet here is the book he has written, having somehow decided not to die. You are reading a book written by a dead man.

I grieved for Martino when I saw that doctor's face. I grieved for the man who had been a friend so highly valued that I couldn't conceive how to pay the emotional price when the bill arrived that day. Alone in a funereal cubicle, I made the vertiginous adjustment. A man who would always put me first, always find solutions to my problems, always deal with the maelstrom in my head, had been suddenly recast as the centre of the universe. Like we shared a brain and his took the bullet.

In the years that followed I watched with wonder as Tino repaired the tissue in his mind, learned to live without being able to read, lost his marriage, underwent brain surgery while awake (for fuck's sake!?), went from a highly cultured, over-educated, five-language-speaking, three-degrees-in-everything, having an encyclopaedia of opinions on communism, sculpture, movies, Cuba, opera, the whole damn shebang, to a gentle, mindful shaman quietly watching with a light beyond words in his eyes. Plus he wrote a book, this book.

The book is excellent, of course. Way beyond cancer porn, it's weird and insightful and is kind of like a guidebook for people who find themselves alive after they've died.

That day, that doctor's face, alone in that cubicle, that was the last time I cried. Now whenever I see Martino I am reminded of how little I know of life and death, how little I know of anything, compared to him. How we don't know what is within us or what may lie on the other side. I have always believed there's something. More than ever after what Tino has done. I hope it's as magical and beautiful as this book, written by a dead man.

Russell Brand, 2016

Preface

A tragicomic memoir about surviving impossible odds,
written by a man who cannot read.

I have written this whole book without ever reading a sentence of it. Words do appear on screen as I am typing away, but upon trying to read them, something funky happens. This is not a conceptual art piece, it's just my new reality, and I'm trying to come to terms with it by writing this book.

The whole idea seemed mad to me at the beginning, and it continued to feel like that until chapter nineteen, when I realized that I had almost reached the end.

I have made peace with the fact that every word I type has to pass through the magnetic tongue of 'Alex', the computer voice that never gets tired of reading back to me my endless mistakes. Fortunately, Alex has no ego and there are no unions in China, where he was created, so I have been able to narrate my lurid tale in the first person, and not as a continuous comedic double act. After all, from its very inception, this book was supposed to be an enlightening and, I hope, inspiring story.

It is almost exactly five years since I was told that I had a ninety-eight per cent chance of dying within eighteen months, and when I kept finding those numbers being substantiated on the internet, my view of reality and its falsifiable religion shifted quite radically – as did my character and my emotions.

The fact that I have used all the tricks that are allowed, some that aren't yet allowed and others that many say have no relevance whatsoever to my health, means that it is now impossible to discern what is actually keeping the aggressive eukaryotic cells that have squatted in my head (or Aliens, as I like to call them), at bay.

I have been told that in one of the most esteemed oncology magazines there is an article about how well my brain is doing, and I do hope that at the end, in the acknowledgements, they haven't forgotten to give some credit to all my own relevant contributions (from my discussions during the brain surgery I underwent while awake, to my adventures in vegan cuisine).

I have no doubt that writing this book saved my life in many different ways. I don't mean philosophically: I really do consider the work that I have been doing with Alex on this computer every day for years to be an essential part of my oncological explorations.

Before all of this, my 'normal' everyday communication with the human beings around me was done mainly through conversations about what we had all read, be it books, articles or someone else's treatments and screenplays. And for me, the words in a treatment or screenplay were always essential. I would judge writers on the basis of such details.

While one must obey the standard industry lexicon when presenting things like 'The camera tracks the night sky – A SEARCHLIGHT floods the LENS', the verbal configuration of a character's dialogue is a true art. It is what defines and makes us love Tarantino's horrible characters. For example, while reading good dialogue, I would automatically get inside the head of a character and the way he lived his life. By page five, a good screenplay would draw me into the rhythm of the language, and the speed of the words with their slight breaks, and make me forget that I was reading. I would be *in* the story.

I do vaguely remember deciding what was the right word or structure of a phrase by re-reading the previous sentence and getting the 'mood' right. But now in this new reality, when I try to edit the text with Alex's voice, I am aware that my decisions are insecure. When I try to 'read' even the best character dialogues, all the energy is pulled out. I have to accept the approximation of my emotions, as I will never again be able to know how a normal reader will react to the words I have written. But I resolved that the only physical way in which I could fight to remain alive was to confront my demons, my inability to read, head on.

In the summer of 2016, after a good couple of years of not really speaking to each other properly, my wife Margarita and I found ourselves sitting together in a restaurant in her home town of Skopje, Macedonia. As the sounds of traditional Slav music shielded us from the otherwise completely empty garden, we finally started talking about the story that has taken place in the past five years and that, with the help of Alex, I have represented in this book. Time had passed and we allowed ourselves to talk about the battles that she and the rest of my family had fought on my behalf to keep me alive and how it has inevitably had an emotional impact on herself and our marriage. Afterwards, as I inserted Margarita's thoughts and feelings into the footnotes throughout the book, I realized how radically narratives and perspectives can change and differ, and how during this tale my own ego had slowly but surely come to the forefront.

My relationship with my type of cancer, which even after its fifth birthday does not allow me to use the word 'remission', has now finally found a place in my daily life. I am aware that the strange, oncological time machine that is in my head will never disappear, but I have also gained a calm and humble appreciation of having survived up to now.

Recently, I even found myself distractedly imagining our eight-year-old boy as a teenager, chatting up girls – something that I had thought time would never allow me to do.

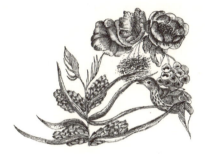

1

A Hole in My Book

How would you feel if you knew that this book, the one that I am writing for you now, was going to be the last book you will ever read? That the curious movement of your well-trained brain will, quite naturally, put these words one after the other, until the day when you fall asleep and wake up with a hole in your head, a gap in your brain, exactly where text is interpreted as words, where memory joins letters together so as to recognize them as consecutive parts of sentences.

One of the great advantages of my current situation is that posters, those sheets of paper that try to influence our desires

5

on the street or on public transport, no longer have any kind of subliminal power over me. While a part of your brain might be stashing away information about the cars you should be driving, the type of food that is essential to your children's growth, or the movies that you should watch, I am free to wander through that world with my own private, healthy predilections. Sadly though, it is exactly the same pure, clean affiliation with text that makes my relationship with books and bookshops so tense these days.

At some point, you must have clicked on one of those gigantic websites, skimmed through the various alternatives that were being suggested to you by your computer, which by now knows exactly what kind of story you need for this month, this weather, or this phase of your life, and you will have managed to get through all the series of five-star reviews from people whose lives and tastes are supposed to be somehow equivalent to yours, and ended up choosing this book that I am writing for you.

When I try to look at those sites, I find that there are too many words in different parts of that endless scrolling page and, not managing to highlight the right parts to be read back to me, I end up fighting with the machine. Occasionally I still find myself walking into old-school bookshops and wandering instinctively towards the areas where, at some point, I must have discovered some treasures, until I suddenly realize the daftness of that endeavour and the sadness of not coming to terms with my new reality.

To overcome my embarrassment, to justify my forgetfulness, I look around for the colourful children's department, pick something up and act as if I am reading it. I ask advice from mothers who seem to have boys of four or five years old, and confused by their kind suggestions, which I know I will never find amongst all those bookcases, I get yet another Dr Seuss story, whose packaging I can recognize from afar.

It may be that you found yourself clicking on this book

because you were attracted by the artful design on the cover, and then became intrigued by the idea of a book co-written by a computer voice. But whilst attempting to write it, I realize that I am now closer to 'Alex', the male voice of this computer, than to any human being. Every sentence that I write, I give to Alex. He reads me the text and reminds me coldly of my poor spelling, my diminished vocabulary, and my not having a memory for names or words.

Let me give you a quick description of the sequence I follow in writing a book with him. Holding my right thumb firmly on the metal square below the spacebar of my laptop, I move my index finger from the beginning of the sentence down towards the end of the page, and as my selected text is covered by the light blue strips, I let go. I look at that artistically designed shape and as my left hand presses my thumb on the 'Ctrl', my index finger quickly follows on the 'S' button, releasing Alex's voice into the world.

I have set up a medium speed for his voice, to give me time to stop him by pressing 'Ctrl' and 'S' again. I always keep my left hand on that stop. If Alex continues reading, I lose track of what I needed to change. Sadly, he hasn't yet learned my particular writing style.

These are some of the words that both Alex and I get wrong:

Red vs Read
Seam vs Seem
Site vs Sight
Whole vs Hole
Warm vs Worm
Sun vs Son
Year vs Ear
Loose vs Lose
Heard vs Herd
Right vs Write
None vs Nun

Right now, as I do not have a physical relationship with anyone, my marriage has collapsed, and my meetings about European films are mostly done through Skype, Alex is the only one that goes to bed with me and reads me newspaper articles. In exactly the same tone, he narrates all the emails that have been sent to me, including the angry language that my wife sometimes uses, when, for whatever reason, she is in a bad mood. At times, he surprises me by reading, in exactly the same male American accent, the love letters that she also writes to me when she is in a good mood.

What can I say? I do have other relationships with other voices in my iPod or iPad, and Alex doesn't really mind. In his free time he meditates together with both his German and Italian friends, who take over his job when I am supposed to read text in those other languages. None of them are ever jealous, which I kind of miss, as it is exactly that instinctive sense of protectiveness that could keep me excited. My assumption is that emotions are crucial parts of communication, but, for now, I guess, Alex and I will have to accept reality as it is, and tell you this story with his voice, and my fingers tapping away on my com-pu-ter.

Thank you, Alex, for not reminding me of the ridiculous words and mistakes that I constantly make. The human world is already very good at doing that, and I certainly need calm to fight this battle.

It was probably my relationship with Alex that made you decide this book was going to be a bit more fun than the thriller you were reading this time last year, and so you purchased *The Finch in My Brain* with certain expectations.

You are probably curious to figure out how, and why, your narrator has stopped being able to read, and why he is actually still alive. I will attempt to answer all your questions, but please be patient, as this is a rather complex journey for me to undertake. While some of this tale is written in the first person, present tense, you'll see that other parts are more classically in the past tense. I do promise that, in time, each part in its own way will be revealed, so, here we go . . .

Los Angeles, 18 January 2011

Lub . . . dub . . . thump thump, ba boom, ba bump, lub-dub ba-dum, ba-dum, ba-dum-tsh, what is this?

Is it English?

Tup tup, tup tup, tup tup – at times it sounds Slav . . . or am I hearing ba-dumm, bumm bumm, poch poch, right now? It sounds like . . . Bavarian? Or maybe it's closer to the Italian tu tump, bom bom, poum poum, bpaum paum, which no, actually now feels . . . yes, more Parisian. It is always exactly the same beat, so why do I now feel that I am having a güm güm, küt küt, güm güm sound sensation that reminds me of . . . Istanbul?

What is happening? What place is this beat trying to remind me of? Where am I? 'Ooh, aah, phew!' I rub my eyes and slowly try to get my bearings. The fact that I do not recognize the white, industrial-looking ceiling above me implies that I am not waking up from a dream, in any place or country I know. I have the feeling that whatever just happened, well . . . it must have been more than a little bit intense.

I do recognize this continuous background sound, but I don't remember from where or when. I must have heard it . . . Yes, God . . . here it is. I have cables that hang down on my arms from both sides and machines constantly beeping away. Their repetition of this sound is here to remind me that I am alive, while somehow the opposite could be true.

As I slowly move my head towards the left, I encounter the huge brown eyes of my wife, Margarita. With her brown hair tied loosely at the back, she is as beautiful as ever. She smiles and looks tired, as if she has not slept for a long time.*

As she gets closer to me, I feel overwhelmed by these wonderful beats of my heart. I don't think I have ever sat listening to the sound of my blood beating. It is probably always the same, but for me, for this moment, and for the view of my wife who has evidently crossed the world to be here, that beat is bliss. The number one in the charts. A little robotic machine and its buzzing sound. Ringo Starr, Keith Moon or Max Roach . . . no matter where they are, they could not drum any better than this.

While entranced by that rhythm, I feel my wife's hand touch mine. That skin, which I almost recognize as my own, transfuses a whole cluster of her emotions on to me. I am still not clear about where I am, or what has happened, and start to feel overwhelmed by the movement of my own smile. I feel happy, really and purely happy, and I am not sure why. I look at Margarita and the first words that come out of my mouth are, 'I could never get you to come and live in London, and now I've got you across the world to Los Angeles!'†

As she tries to hug me, I notice that she is moving her arms in an awkward way. My head seems covered with what feels like a puffy winter hat. Behind her shoulders I see the white hair of my mother, Marianella, who is holding a sheet of typed paper in her hands that she seems to be scanning intently. A pose I have often observed, when she has been standing in front of her endless rows of books in her house in Milan.

---

* Margarita Sclavi: 'Before I walked into your room in the hospital, everyone from the nurses to the doctors simply threw pieces of dreadful information at me. Somehow assuming, as I was a doctor, that I could understand it all.'

† Margarita: 'I remember walking into your room wearing a leather jacket and my blue and white striped shirt. No one else was in the room and as you were trying to be funny, I looked into your eyes, and understood that they were no longer your eyes. Even if I was finally there, next to you, emotionally you were somewhere else. There was a layer between us, a coldness . . . that has never gone away.'

Next to her, with an almost silly smile and waving her hand back and forth, there is my big sister, Bianca, who lives in a lovely flat in Paris. I am lying at centre stage and from here I have somehow galvanized a family reunion. I guess that all three of them have been forced to enter into my new, alternative reality, whatever that is.

This is all a bit too intense. Even though I have just woken up, I feel tired, I feel I urgently need to sleep a tiny bit more. I close my eyes and hope that, at some point, when I wake up, someone will tell me what exactly has happened to my head and why I don't seem to remember anything . . .

～

Is it a different day? Or have they all left me to nap? I seem to be high up, around the twentieth floor, in a corner room. The design of this place is actually quite cool. It is like the set of a science fiction film. When I look out of the window, I see a big church surrounded by a huge, empty parking lot. Yes, I am in LA, and here everybody needs a car to go and pray. But why is it always empty? When do they go to church? What day is it? That architecture is not similar to any church I know. It must be . . . oh yes, it is the church of L. Ron Hubbard. I am lying on a hospital bed opposite the Church of Scientology. God, should I be looking at them for my salvation?

That makes sense. American healthy competition. Where there is a McDonald's, you must have a Burger King, a KFC, or at the very least a Domino's Pizza. So, you can choose. Scientology or hospitals? Scientology does slightly scare me, but so does the cut that the hospital has made on my head. I hope I am on the right side of the street.

There are so many religions and right now I could genuinely use one. I have to lean on some belief system. Something really strong that can hold my brain steady. Sorry, God. Really, really sorry. I know I've not visited you in church very often – or at all in the last twenty years. I guess that coming to see the beautiful art and architecture that you have inspired in your churches does not count, and now that I've apparently been cut to bits, the only church I have next to me is Scientology, and as far as they are concerned, I am definitely talking with the wrong God.

A few months ago, while sitting outside the Indian embassy in Rome, I humoured my friend Matteo, who has recently enrolled in tantric yoga classes, and I started reading a book he gave me, whose name I do not remember. It described how both Buddhist and Vedic traditions are deeply committed to the idea of out-of-body experiences, reincarnation and near-death episodes. Well, those hippy spiritual happenings that I read about in that book? I think I just had one of those.

From what I remember, these events originate in a brain, right while it is shutting down. Their role is to help us accept and embrace our death, or maybe in this case they were just my private drunken tourist guides, helping me ride my own Nautilus back to this hospital in Los Angeles.

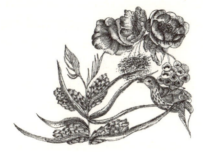

2

Operational Glamorama

Los Angeles, 20 January 2011

It is visiting hour and the first person I see walking into my huge single room is my mother, Marianella, who seems to have become taller than my friend Russell Brand, who is trailing behind her along with all the lads of his entourage. As she gets closer to me, her glasses hanging down on their strings, I notice that her short white hair has grown. The smile on her face seems extremely tense, almost as if she were grinding her teeth.

She grabs my hand and says, 'You look great with this new haircut.'

I reply, 'I'm told they cut out a piece of my brain and I feel fine. I guess I didn't really need it.'

I know that when Marianella is focused on one thing she manages to forget everything else that is happening in the world, and as she often admits, she frequently ends up burning coffee or even boiled eggs. I remember once as a little kid playing in the sand on the beach at Rimini, where she grew up, and after seeing her swim away in the sea, I waited for what seemed forever and made peace with the fact that she had forgotten all about me.

It is extremely aggravating for me right now not to be able to answer any of her endless questions about what happened last night. I am conscious that someone has cut out a part of my brain; the puffy material surrounding my head confirms it. But I really do not know what to say and as the mood in this room is quite tense, I turn my eyes towards Russell, expecting him to pull out from his well-trained head one of his sharp, witty elucidations of events. But I guess I have caught him off guard . . . I don't think I have ever seen him searching for words before.

His assistant, Tom Chadwick, gives a little smile and steps towards me to fill the gap.

'Do you remember? As we were preparing for Russ's show, you lay down and slept on that big couch by the entrance. We were all concerned, because you had been telling us about the headaches that were going all the way down to your nose. I woke you up as your friend Kenneth Francis arrived at the door, and you told me that he was going to help you find a doctor. You seemed sure that with a few pills and a bit of sleep everything was going to sort itself out.'

I feel as if I am in a science fiction film, where the other characters are speaking in a different language. Or perhaps it's just me who is confusing time, space and perspective:

Me: 'And then what happened?'

Nicola, Russell's lovely and always so calming hair and makeup lady, looking at Tom: 'There at the theatre, as we started moving towards the stage, your phone . . .'

Tom, nodding his head: 'Yes, my phone was buzzing in my pocket, so I moved away,' and looking at Russell, 'It was just as you were about to step on stage.'

Russell stares at Tom, shrugs his shoulders in a sign of absolutely no recollection. I am glad that I am not the only person here feeling as if I am listening to a piece of fiction.

Now Tom is talking: 'The call was from your phone, so I was quite surprised to hear a female voice on the other end. It was a nurse from the ER, who had found the phone in the pocket of your jacket and I guess had just pressed the last number called. When I got to the hospital, your friend was not there and the nurse told me that when she started her shift you were already lying down on a bed sleeping all alone.'

Me: 'I really don't remember any of this. If my friend told those nurses about the pain I had been having in my nose . . . they must have just assumed that I was a passed-out cokehead.'

Nicola, still with five hair grips stuck on her shirt from doing Russell's hair: 'Tom's calls from the hospital sounded quite scary,' and looking at Russell, 'and somehow even the show didn't seem to flow very well.'

Tom looks at me almost apologetically.

Nicola, now facing me: 'As soon as Russ came off stage, we all got into the car and came over here to see what was happening.'

Russell, with his hand on my mother's shoulder: 'The doc told us that it was looking really bad and explained that you weren't waking up because there was something putting a lot of pressure on your brain. They needed to operate . . . right away. As a nurse was giving you an injection, the doc told me that he was waking you up. It only took a few seconds, you opened your eyes – and you were back amongst us . . .'

Tom: 'You were totally awake and very confused.'

Russell: 'I tried to tell you what was going on, but you weren't really clear about where you were or what was happening to you.'

After a pause, Tom: 'It was quite scary.'

Even as their voices continue, I get lost looking at the ceiling of the room. Am I in a film? The set does look perfect, and so is the lighting. All these characters are talking and looking at me, but I seem to have lost the sound somewhere. This is one of those conceptual art shows, right? Fritz Lang's *Metropolis* was mute, wasn't it? Like this, that one also had a mad doctor and a robotic machine.

Am I supposed to come out enlightened? What are they all doing here? What are they talking about? My mother's face is captivated by Tom. She is definitely more engaged in the story than I am.

A nurse enters the room with a bunch of plastic bottles, so I raise my hand to Tom to tell him to wait a minute as I ask her, 'Sorry, I feel something very uncomfortable here. Can one of you help me . . . take it out?'

I guess I haven't expressed myself clearly. I smile at her. She is now looking at me, confused.

'I don't know exactly what happened in my head or to what extent my brain has been cut open, but I am pretty sure that whatever it is, it has nothing to do with this rubber bag covering my penis right now, has it? I tried, but I can't manage to take it out.'

She stops what she is doing, looks me straight in the eye, shakes her head and says, 'No.'

Before openly starting to beg her, I try using my old charm, if I still have any . . .

'Come on, it's like wearing a heavy wool sweater at the beach. So can you please, pretty please, help me take it out? I really do need things to make sense. And I don't think this thing makes any sense at all. Please, I need to pee. Can you help me?'

She is checking if the liquid is trickling down properly from the bottle that she has just replaced up there and, almost rhythmically, she pulls out one of the big bags hanging below me. She smiles and, looking behind her at the various people around my bed, says, 'Honey, you know you were a very bad boy last night? When I came to prepare you for the operation and tried to insert the catheter . . . well, you started to get violent with me.'

I look at her, stunned, not really sure if I want to hear the rest of her story.

'I brought in two other nurses with me, but we still couldn't hold you fast.'

She moves her eyes towards Russell, urging him to continue the tale, but he coyly looks away. He doesn't seem to want to tell me this story. He says cautiously, 'Mate, you don't remember *any* of this?'

I shake my head, surprised, and intrigued to hear some more from him.

'I tried to get you to calm down, and explained why this

thing was necessary, but you didn't seem to care about anything. Even when I told you that they were preparing you for brain surgery! You just didn't want them to stick that thing in your dick . . . which I totally understood.' He looks at the nurse again with a knowing half-smile and adds, 'I was trying to help them by holding your arms back and keeping you distracted.'

Now he hesitates and the nurse tells me, 'Yes, you bit him. Really hard on the arm. Several times.'

Russell, half-laughing, says, 'I just gave up. You did not want that thing in your dick and I couldn't do anything about it. I just told them to let you piss yourself.'

'Wow, really? Why don't I remember any of this? I kind of feel guilty . . . Sorry.' Then, with my hand on the plastic sack, I add, 'I guess that I was defeated in the end last night, but *now* can you take it away?'

A young man in a white coat appears at the door.

Russell gets up close and tells me, 'He's your doc, the guy who cut your head open last night. He is a very nice guy, you'll like him.' Raising his hand towards him, 'Hello, doc!'

The surgeon looks straight at me with a warm smile, as though nobody else were in the room. 'Hello, I am Doctor Vogel, how are you feeling?'

I smile back at him, move my shoulders up from the pillow to show him the back of my head, as if to say, what do you think? He touches the fabric covering my head, folds in a little part that is covering the top of my left eye, and looks very satisfied. Even if everybody in the room looks cheery, I feel like this pause is too long. I want to know more from him.

As his eyes properly meet mine, I realize that there is more communication in that man-to-man physical contact than any dialogue that I have ever had. There is nothing simpler than the story of a doctor who saves a life. There is no question about it. With no Vogel, there would be no story, no book and no hope for a happy ending. So, let's get on with this.

From the other side of my bed, Russell says, 'There was this lady from the management staff who walked up to me while we' – he points to the doctor – 'were talking last night. She somehow thought I was next of kin or, in any case, the person who she should be asking for money. Not having found any proof of your insurance, she actually tried to have a discussion with me about money. I understand that she has a shit job, but the only thing I could tell her was, "Do you think that this is the moment to talk money? I'm talking to the doctor here about you dying, and you want *money*? We're in the ER, where money should *not* be the top emergency!"'

Dr Vogel nods and says, 'It was good that you stayed here.' I look at him, confused. He continues, 'If you'd had a similar experience at one of the hospitals for no-income patients, well, I don't think you would be alive now.'

'That wasn't the only argument of the night,' Russell adds. 'Before the operation, you had an animated discussion with the doc.' Dr Vogel smiles. 'You said it's not fair to have a country without National Health Care . . . and as they were cutting your hair off, you got proper angry, and continued your rant about "Everybody should do something about that!" And the doc kept saying "Right" to calm you down.'

This time the doctor interjects, saying 'Right!' again with a smile. And I wonder if he is just backing Russell's story or is he actually supporting my political view? Whatever. In any case, this is the first bit of the story that does not surprise me.

Russell's enormous but gentle bodyguard sees that we are in a good mood and chips in, 'It wasn't enough that you had no health insurance, you were also talking like a commie!', which makes everybody laugh.

Russell continues, 'This other lady told me that I had to call your next of kin to get their approval for the operation. So I called Margarita a few times, but she didn't answer. So I called your sister, who I guess called your mother. Even if we finally got Margarita and Miro on a plane, the doctors couldn't wait.'

He puts his hand on mine. 'I looked the doc in the eyes

before he took you away and told him to please take care and make sure to bring you back alive. And please not to cut away the bits of your brain that you were going to still need to continue making our big revolutionary films.'

'So who ended up signing the paperwork for me?'

~

At least inside this book, I have to make sure that everything continues to be clear. Even if I have never written one of these things before, I am pretty sure that some of the structural parts of it must be similar to the Hollywood films that you like. See, here I am trying to establish the stakes right at the beginning and engaging you with the human side of the story.

In this chapter it is 2011, and I just have to keep in mind (which is no easy task given the fact that I forget almost everything, and there is not yet a computer that can help me with this) that your experience, while reading this book, should be emotional, enticing, exciting . . . and a bunch of other words starting with E.

In order to do this, let me begin writing in the past tense. The present is a bit too arduous – at least for me – right now. Occasionally I will snap back to this present, at times a little, at times a lot, and by so doing I will hopefully inject some fresh air, some fun parts, that will escort you (and me) all the way to the end.

~

Russell's crew gave Margarita, Bianca and my mother everything they could possibly need: US mobile phones, pyjamas, socks, toothbrushes, beauty products and a gigantic quantity of toys for our two-year-old son Miro. They organized a room in the hospital for the family a few floors down from me, so they could take turns staying with Miro and coming up to see me.

After a few days, I was moved from intensive care to a regular room and Bianca and Marianella showed me that among the various gifts I had received of sweets, flowers and books, there was also a doggy bag containing all my hair. In the emotion of the operation, Russell had told the nurses that perhaps I would like to keep it. We cheerfully tried to imagine what I could do with it as a reminder of our time in that Californian hospital. We could sew it together and make a scarf, a man bag for my telephone, a wig for my skull, a cushion for my naps, or even a symbolic brooch to pin on the breast pocket of my jacket.*

Our light-hearted, good-humoured family meeting was interrupted by the entrance of a young woman doctor with a cold professional attitude. She was one of the oncology assistants. Little well-mannered smiles and evasive eyes. I thought she had come in to see how I was doing. My mother, Marianella, is a highly regarded expert in 'conflict resolution' and people in Italy love the books that she writes. She is continuously invited to give lectures in every part of the country on how to negotiate conflicts in companies, towns or schools. Now, with her professorial tone of voice, she asked, 'Do you know what he has? And more precisely, what caused this attack?'

The young assistant had the biopsy results in her hand and she had come precisely to communicate them to us.

'He has a grade-four glioblastoma.'

My mother asked her to please translate this into everyday language. 'What is that?'

'It's a very aggressive form of cancer. Grade four is the most violent of them all.'

I tried to focus and make my brain follow this discussion. There were so many strange words, so many raw emotions floating in the room that I somehow lost my way.

My eyes were working fine. I saw every detail of those faces, but the sound disappeared from my screen. As my mother's face tensed up with anger, she raised her arms, opened both

---

* Margarita: 'As I arrived at the hospital, I asked the nurses and everyone else if I could have your hair. But they did not give it to me. For me it was precious. I wanted the hair of your old life.'

of her hands and glared at the young doctor, as if she were a wicked little rat running aimlessly around in the room.

In that moment, I did not care about the audio. All the information that I needed to take in was playing itself out right in front of me. It was not the hyper reality of a mute sci-fi film, quite the opposite; it was . . . extremely . . . real.

My sister's expression was equally shocked. She put her hands on my mother's shoulder, not so much for moral support, as to make sure that she would not take that doctor creature in her hands and squeeze her soul out of her throat. I looked at her calmly, as an un-engaged spectator, and told her, 'I guess you must be accustomed to this kind of reaction . . . but you have just stepped on the wrong Italian mother.'

She walked quickly out of the room and left Bianca and me to deal with our mother's wrath.

~

The reason I could not fully engage with what was happening in that hospital room was because of a precise, historical moment that I have tattooed in my memory. I had seen my mother in that state only once before, when I was twenty-five years old. I had come back from Cambridge University to visit my father, who was in a six-person room in the main hospital of Milan. He had been sick for a year, but none of the high-ranking professors really understood what he had and what they could do about it.

One day, my father was lying in his hospital bed, with his usual copies of *The Economist* and the *New Yorker* next to him, while various doctors in front of him were conferring about how bad his illness was. They did so without ever looking him in the eye, and so treated him like an animal in a stall, or at the very least an idiot who couldn't really understand their complex discussions.

When their dialogue had reached its zenith, and their faces had tightened as a sign of having given up, they turned around to walk out, only to find the door blocked by the body of

Marianella, who verbally burned their arrogant white coats and forced them to stand naked in front of my father and tell him that they were impotent and lost and to apologize for their attitude. On that occasion, neither Bianca nor I held her back and we never saw those doctors again.

I spent a morning talking to my father about the strange dreams he was having. He told me that during the night he had imagined being in the midst of a game of Pac-Man, where he had to run away from creatures that were chasing him from all sides. At the end of his tale, he told me to go home and sleep, as I had spent the whole night there and he was, anyway, tired and needed to take a nap. That was the last time I saw him. As soon as I arrived home and lay down on the bed, the phone rang and a friend of his told me to come back to the hospital, as my father needed my help. When I arrived, he was already dead. From then on, he has stayed with me, and accompanied me as my spiritual Jedi Master.

At night, when it's calm and silent here in this American hospital, I often find myself talking to my father Gastone, and I ask him for advice or try to make him smile.

'Dad, isn't it weird that my first encounter with the Aliens has taken place in, of all obvious locations for a film producer, Los Angeles? I never thought I would end up in this town, with their hippy drinks and even stranger religions. Up to now, I've never made any effort to enter their rich world and I've always assumed that they wouldn't be interested in my "European" kind of storytelling.'

My father does not seem to have any problem with my tale of the Aliens and, silently, he asks me to tell him more.

'You know, as a young boy, when I would walk to the bathroom in the middle of the night to pee, I'd often see you sitting in bed with the light on and a book in your hands. Thrillers, biographies, politics, economics or historical analyses, you just seemed to churn through every type of book. Even if your legacy as a leader of the unions has obviously influenced many of the decisions that I've made in my life, I know that at heart you have always been a scientist.

'I remember when I was six and I asked you for a gun, and you sat me down on the couch with you, and with a piece of paper and a pen, you explained to me exactly how a bullet is placed in a gun, and where and how the energy is released so powerfully that the bullet comes out with enough strength to fracture a human body and take a life away. The result was that I no longer wanted to hold a gun. You broke down even the most complex science into an understandable language, a gift that fortunately Bianca has inherited from you. So, I am sure that you'll understand my current technical problem with Aliens. I am feeling the attack, Dad, and I guess it's like your old-school Pac-Man video game. I don't have enough energy right now to understand what their ultimate aim is in this game, but talking about it has calmed me down. Thanks.'

~

I had to decide if I wanted my son Miro to come to my hospital room the next day so that we could celebrate his third birthday together. I really needed to hug him and I asked everybody to make this happen, if at all possible. We studied different ways in which I could cover my head so as not to scare him. How we could organize the room in a way that it would look . . . child-friendly. And who else could we invite? Would other children be able to come in here?

We tried. We really did try, but it was impossible. There was no way to render that space less scary to a small child who had just flown across the world to find his father, so we gave up.

Margarita told me that they had organized the most memorable children's party at Russell Brand and Katy Perry's house, but even though the living room was filled with toys of all kinds, balloons, music and songs, Miro was jet-lagged and did not want to play. She had tried to introduce him to his new friends and showed him all his toys, but he just refused it all and insisted on going back to bed, leaving everyone in a birthday party without a birthday boy.

Miro, like most children, is happy to re-watch the same film over and over, and every time he seems just as surprised and excited. In that period, aged two to three, there were some films that he was addicted to and it was largely my fault. Every time I came back from London I would bring Miro either a small Thomas the Tank Engine train, or a new DVD of *Thomas and Friends*. As part of my attempt to make him grow up speaking English in Italy, I allowed him to watch more of those films than I normally would have.

There was a film that had accompanied me throughout my time at Cambridge that I guess I was also addicted to. It was called *Gattaca*, written and directed by Andrew Niccol, starring Ethan Hawke, Uma Thurman and Jude Law. It was set in a near future where parents conceived children through a computer. This guaranteed them an unsurpassable output, by mixing together the best parts of both DNAs. In fact, the central religion of those doctors was science. Anything that a scientific study told them, that was the truth.

In this story the Ethan Hawke character is one of the few remaining people to have been conceived naturally, and so, compared with most others, including his brother, he is inferior. Having grown up with this sad predicament, the main aim of his life is to prove the whole scientific world wrong.

I guess we didn't have much to do in Cambridge, because my American friend Emily James and I must have watched the film several times, and when we weren't watching it, we were probably in a pub talking about its wider implications.

Now that I was lying in a hospital bed in Los Angeles, the land of stories and cinema, and had just been given my life expectancy results from a doctor, I had myself entered the world of *Gattaca*. In every way possible, I had to get around it. I had a ninety-eight per cent chance of dying in the next year and a half, which meant that I still had a three per cent chance of survival – of cracking the code of this scientific religion – of showing them all that their paradigm is collapsing, and that I will confound all their expectations and post the new recipe for free on Pinterest, Twitter, Facebook, YouTube and whatever else they come up with.

But before I can do that, I need a strategy, a plan, or just a better understanding of what is actually happening in this story.

~

From the moment when Russell decided to stay here with us and not go to a big, glamorous show in London, where he was due to receive an award for Outstanding Contribution to British Comedy, the press has turned its powerful eyes in my direction and in every newspaper there seem to be stories of how he has remained in LA to stay near his friend.

I have just read an article where they have published a photo of my boy Miro being carried on Russell's shoulders into this very place. They both have a hospital sticker on their T-shirts and my boy looks happy. There are people from the hospital that I have never seen who now pass by and smile at me. Everybody who comes into my room shows me articles on their phones or computers. (Yes, I only lost my ability to read after the second operation, the one done while I was awake. We'll come to that.)

I have never really followed Russell and Katy's relationship with the media. While they are used to dealing with it on a daily basis, and have somehow made peace with it, for me this is just strange. How did the press get to know that 'Sclavi had complained of "searing headaches" on Wednesday' or that 'Sclavi is in a critical condition'? I know that some of that is probably correctly quoted, as most definitely is also the bit that they pulled out of Russell's autobiography *My Booky Wook*, where he talks about me as if I were 'an exceptional man', by whom he 'always felt encouraged and protected', but, sadly in that very same article they say that we are in a hospital in New York City. This may seem a small detail to you, but it brings me right back to my essential problem – isn't all narrative (including that of my doctors in this hospital) falsifiable?

I am lying here in this hospital bed and getting more press for it than any movie I have put hard work into. It is the commodification of my illness. I smile at this Glamorama surrounding me, but, ultimately, I couldn't care less. Like my son next to his enormous stash of toys, I just want to sleep and hopefully encounter him in my dreams.

～

A few days later I was told I could go home. As my mother and Bianca were there helping me get dressed (I had to be careful while sliding T-shirts over my head), two women in high heels arrived in my room with the printed-out bill in their hands. I owed the hospital $100,000. A nice, clean, abstract number.

They told us that it was 'negotiable', in how and when to pay it. But yes, I had to pay it. The only way to pay a bit less was if I had an American social security number and was low income. I told them that I had lived in America with a Green Card for ten years and that, somehow, I would find my social security number again. All jolly good, but before leaving we had to go downstairs to the financial office and give them a down payment.

We followed them to their tiny office, where my mother pulled out her two Italian credit cards and pointed to the one that was more likely to be useful. The two women took it and asked, 'Can we try to take ten thousand dollars from this?' Our three faces met and almost laughed.

'Sure. Try it,' said my mother. It did not go through, so they tried for five thousand and that did not go through either. They tried two thousand. And still nothing. We did not know what to expect, but we were somehow pleased that the little Italian card did not like them.

Finally they put in one thousand dollars and the card let them have it. Bianca handed over her French card and the operation continued for the remaining two cards before we could walk out of the hospital three thousand dollars poorer. This was definitely going to be an issue, but at least for now, I could go and hug my boy.

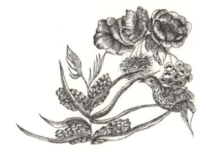

3

The Ten Missing Pages

*This chapter in a Hollywood film would have
'FOUR MONTHS EARLIER' posted on screen as we
see an aeroplane depart. It explains what happened
before the two chapters that you have just read and
how I came to lie in that hospital bed.*

Los Angeles, 2010

My wife Margarita and I were in a plane travelling back to
our lovely apartment in Rome from Jaipur, India, where we

had lived through seven of the most extraordinary days of our lives. There, in our squeezed standard seats, we finally had a moment to talk about what had just happened and how it had pushed us into a parallel reality.

India itself was a radically new experience for both of us, and we were conscious that our first vision of that historical land had been obscured by its glorious packaging. We had just spent a week celebrating the wedding of Russell Brand and Katy Perry at the Aman-i-Khas resort in Rajasthan, Northern India. We had been invited as their guests, along with eighty-five of their friends, to stay with them in a luxury tented camp near a wildlife sanctuary. Looking through the endless photographs, which were going to be essential in describing the surreal events to others, our discussion turned to the main issue of what had occurred earlier that morning.

As everyone was hugging and taking their last pictures before saying their goodbyes, Nik Linnen, Russell's manager and best man, had asked me to walk with him and Russell through the lovely resort which had been hosting us for the past week. There, in the middle of India, accompanied by monkeys and sweeping birds, Russell stopped, stared straight into my eyes and said, 'Come to Los Angeles – we'll create big films and make the revolution there,' smiling at me like a wicked boy who has stolen a ticket to the chocolate factory and wants to share it with me.

Rome, where I was living with my wife and child, was beautiful and the food unequalled, but the economy was collapsing and so the opportunities for work were minimal, and I was desperate to find new adventures. My constant travels and lack of a steady income were a source of tension between Margarita and me. She saw some of our friends around us living 'normal lives', like having a place by the beach to spend the warm summers, and she did not understand why I wasn't finding ways to make that happen.

She is a psychiatrist, one of those fantastic creatures whose profession is to heal others, but if she could, she would much rather spend her time as a painter or interior decorator, not sitting in a room or in a hospital fixing people's brains.

As a teenager she had hung out with many Macedonian film makers and so had already developed her own vision of what my profession looked like. A few years ago, she came with me to the Cannes Film Festival and she definitely liked what she saw. In such situations we did get along fantastically well, and in fact it was there in Cannes that we conceived our boy. So, her question has always been, why don't these trips I take into my glamorous parallel world ever produce anything?

I've tried to empathize with her frustration. Was my job a priority over our relationship? There are people who do manage it, so why couldn't we?

Now, on that aeroplane, with her eyes on all those photos, we talked. Yes, I had been invited to move immediately to LA, where I would help Russell pave his way to superstardom. His new wife was about to start her world tour, which would take her away from him for the good part of a year and a half. Russell needed projects that would keep him busy.

LA was a sixteen-hour flight from Rome and nothing was on paper yet, but somehow I knew that it was going to happen. Even if the scope of our new adventure was not clear, for the first time I could guarantee my wife that some 'proper' money would finally arrive into our bank account. What made this move to LA more feasible was Margarita's new-found friendship with two fantastic Californian ladies: Amanda Fairey, the wife of the American artist Shepard Fairey, and Trina Venit, the wife of Russell's US agent, Adam Venit.

Her new friends were excited by the prospect of having her arrive in their town sometime soon. With their moral and emotional support, I kissed Margarita and jumped on that boat heading for uncharted waters, led by my Jack Sparrow-like friend.

Despite being born in Italy, I had grown up in America and perhaps, after twenty years living in Europe, it was time to rediscover this land of freedom. Our son Miro could grow up in a profoundly different culture, while knowing that when he came back home to Rome, he could kick a ball around and call it 'football'.

From my perspective, I just assumed that this was a pay-off for all my hard, poorly remunerated work so far as a film producer. Margarita now had her LA posse and it seemed like the right moment. We could start expanding our family and giving Miro a few brothers and sisters to play with. I'd produce nice, big, optimistic Hollywood movies, the right thing to do and perhaps the only way in which I could influence society and give meaning to my professional life.

Hope, it seemed to me, was what people were most in need of: hope and trust in themselves and as part of a community. Russell and I would tackle directly the cultural redirection of the world, acting half as story tellers and half as fortune tellers in a film industry where getting rich seemed to be the only legitimate aim.

It sounds good, right?

Russell was still relatively new to the LA habitat and had not yet learnt to drive – a significant problem. Fortunately, he had brought a friend with him from London, who gladly took on the role of chauffeur, since there were rarely moments where his original talent was needed. I had only ever seen this friend at events where he was working as security, and I had absolutely no doubt that if anyone even thought of intruding into Russell's life without permission, he would make sure that they miraculously disappeared from the scene. I am almost six foot three inches tall, and usually see the world from above, but when I am next to him, I stretch my neck and look up at the sky.

As part of Russell's entourage, I lived in a shared house in Los Feliz with his manager Nik Linnen, his assistant Tom, and his bodyguard friend. The first time I landed in LA, I arrived in my little rental car at that empty house and wandered through the rooms, and I found DVDs of the American series *Entourage* lying everywhere. From afar at least, we were all quite stereo-typical in our roles and characters.

A few days after my arrival, Russell, his bodyguard and I travelled to one of the studios (in LA a meeting on the other side of the city is always a journey) to propose some major plot changes for our new film project, *Bad Father*. I had been working intensively on the treatment and we were quite opti-mistic about our new version of the story. I had just entered this world and wanted to let everybody know that Russell's Italian lion was in town.

I knew that the changes I proposed were rather radical, but if we were going to make a big mainstream film, I was going to put in it all the best stuff I had. That included introducing, in some of Russell's scenes set in church, the voice of God (something I had first seen in the black-and-white TV show *Don Camillo*, which my grandmother Luisa loved and used to show me as a child).

If Russell's character had to change throughout this story from a criminal to a saviour, by acting as if he was a priest, he had to have some kind of relationship with God. I ran the idea past Adam Venit, Russell's US agent, and Nik, and they both loved it. The plot was perfect, as was the narrative arc, how could we *not* cast God in our first Hollywood film?

After Russell wittily introduced me to our big producer, Jack Giarraputo, I presented our new story with energy and convic-tion. I was pepped up, and felt that I knew exactly what I was doing. I finished the narration of the third act, with our completely new 'socially optimistic' ending, and looked at him with a smile. Even before my smirk could leave my face, Jack shook his head and, with extreme efficiency and clarity, knocked it down. He had read the document that I had sent him that morning and knew that none of it was necessary.

As far as he was concerned, the script that already existed was good enough and no God, or other revolutionary ideas I was presenting, would change what was for them a strong film going into production. Russell and I, like eagerly confident teenagers, tried to defend our arguments, but shortly afterwards accepted the retreat and found the positive sides in the existing treatment, as the big studio boss was suggesting.

Jack, who has produced all of Adam Sandler's films, recapped for us which kind of story had made what kind of money. There was no doubt that he knew how to make money. At that moment at least, his financial credibility managed to overwhelm the obvious difference between his conservative political philosophy and our rather radical, revolutionary aims. Reconstructing and finishing the story by showing the audience that we can all change, and make a better world, was in no way an economic priority for him.

Finally, he gave us one of his writers and we were off. So, the story that I had to make peace with started with a small-time crook (Russell), who was about to be killed by a bunch of gangsters, having tried to sell them a set of fake credit cards. Through pure serendipity, our protagonist takes refuge in a small, very Catholic town, in the middle of nowhere, where he starts acting as the new priest.

Even if it was not what I originally wanted, I was sure that I could create something that would make us all happy. I soon realized that stepping on the ego of such a successful producer was not going to get me anywhere.

Paul Berbaum, the scriptwriter, and I met initially in the house in Los Feliz. It was a fenced-in neighbourhood that offered great calm. Crucially, we had an outside terrace where I could smoke while talking to Paul inside. Nik, Russell's bodyguard and Tom were almost never there in the mornings when we met. Those days I went out early, had a coffee in a bar nearby, and picked up croissants for the both of us. Sadly, that lovely rhythm only lasted until the day when Paul, Russell and I went up to the studios to meet the producer and talk through the first act.

Jack Giarraputo had a big office space, its walls covered in posters of the countless films he had produced with Adam

Sandler. But during any shooting there in the lot, he always stayed in his trailer, only two hundred yards from his office. He was very proud of his trailer, and even more of the fried steaks and eggs that he cooked up during the meeting. No matter how rich he was, he still seemed to like his caravan more than anything else, and while he was eating his food, we presented our work to him.

We had made some minor changes that I hoped would drive the story a bit more in my original direction. I had kept God out of the story, and fortunately, as far as Jack was concerned, it was all good. I assumed that he hadn't read the last version of the script recently, but I was immediately surprised that he not only spotted our little changes, but he also remembered variations that had been made six months before. The man was sharp and obviously on top of his game and, for me, that somehow justified his wealth, which I guess had come from having made lots of people laugh.

He suggested that we shoot the film in Las Vegas, the gambling capital of America. As well as having some financial incentives for the producers, it was an exciting place in which to set the story, though our cheating priest would still be hiding up in a nearby small town. We discussed the timing of it and agreed that, due to Russell's other engagements, we should have a draft that the producer could bring to the big studio bosses by mid-January. That was tight, if not impossible, for a whole script, but, hell, I was a tourist in this new land and I guessed I had to play by their rules. If they needed the story ready by then, I would make sure that it was the best it could be, and on time.

Paul had already worked on an old version of *Bad Father* a year before. Jack knew that I had different ideas on how the story should develop, but he trusted Paul and knew that Paul's loyalties lay with him. Paul lived nine hours away from LA, but jumped in a car any time work was calling. Jack paid him a wage and covered the costs of a nearby apartment, but as I had come into the project from Russell's side, he would not be paying me at all.

Paul's apartment was in North Hollywood, so I told him that I would drive up to his neighbourhood to save us a bit of the writing time. I was pushing him to write quickly and I did not want him to be spending half of his day travelling to meet me. The coffee shop he chose for our meetings looked old school. Every table had two wide plastic-covered benches, and all the waitresses had a smile and an attitude. It was 'nearby' in LA distance, which meant forty-five minutes from my house, and ten minutes from his apartment.

I did not mind the trip, especially because I had found bagels (*No, Alex, not beagles*) in that coffee shop. I had bagels every morning, toasted, with cheese, lox and a touch of lemon. It took me back to my New York youth, eating that kind of bread and that kind of breakfast. As page after page of our story developed, I started ordering other things, like pancakes, doughnuts and toasted ham-and-cheese sandwiches.

It was the right diet for the second act, where our unusual priest had surreptitiously started to make the whole little town near Las Vegas fall in love with him. There were no fancy teas in this place, just the type of coffee that they continuously pass by to refill. The one that doesn't taste of anything, but gives better comfort than the quick shot of an espresso. My mouth was warm the whole time and if I really needed it, depending on the scene in discussion, I would even put some sugar in it.

Towards the end of the second act, I stopped ordering food. We had to deliver the script in one week's time and it felt like there was no time to eat. I had not told Paul about the increasing frequency of my powerful headaches. It was maybe only an environmental effect from the smog of this town, or perhaps it was the high stakes that I had set myself for this new job. In any case, I had no time for it. We managed to arrive at the end of the second act with some great set pieces that worked well for both the story arc and the comedy.

Third acts are the trickiest and most financially complex parts of nearly all films. Between the second and third act our main character had to realize that what he had wanted the whole time was actually an illusion, and what was really necessary was for him to make a much bigger leap of faith, and thus save the town and all its picaresque characters.

From the beginning I had been a constant pain for Paul, continuously asking him to stop and make sure that our main character was being truly forced to change, and that we were raising the stakes in every scene in order to surprise and engage the emotions of our audience, but now I started leaving him alone with the material. We had shorter and shorter meetings. A glass of orange juice and that was it. We were working on a possible scene for the third act, which here in Los Angeles would be called the 'Money Shot'.

Actually, the best thing one can do in films like ours is to have three strong endings. You pull out all the gear you've got, and when the audience thinks that they have had enough, that they have hit the zenith of the story, you need to have two more, bigger, funnier, more surprising turns. A triple money shot. Bang . . . Bang . . . Bang! But at that point, I had to tell Paul about my headaches. I had started losing my concentration and finding that I couldn't answer his simple narrative dilemmas, for which, just a week before, I would easily have found a solution.

We had three days before we had to show it to Russell and Nik, so we absolutely had to finish it. The idea was to get everybody who worked in the house to read one of the characters. Tom, Katy's brother, the lovely girl who organized their lives (whose name I unfortunately don't remember and sadly no Alex, Dick or Harry in my computer can help me with that), and a few others that I forget would all be cast for the day. It would take about two and a half hours to read through the whole script. It was our last chance, as Russell and the crew were about to start a three-day stand-up show, which would be filmed for their *Happiness* documentary. After that they were going to New York for an awards ceremony, where Russell was going to pick up some sort of a 'You Are Really Talented' prize.

I left Paul to finish the ending of the story by himself, which made me feel terrible. Throughout the whole journey, and up to that moment, I had been planting in various scenes the seeds for the finale. I had constructed it in such a way that in order for Russell's character to change, he would have to inspire the various people in his small town to be active, to take a stance. Even though I was more than sure that these were going to be the best scenes of the whole film, I just could not do it.

My idea was that over the next few days, as Paul was finishing the third act, I would sleep and look after myself, and then in the next draft, we would get back to the story and change it. By not getting stressed about this, and just being good to my body, I was sure that somehow the headaches would stop.

In the past, headaches had usually only arrived in my head in the mornings, after I'd had a serious drinking adventure the night before. But that was also quite rare for me, even back in my younger days. If I ever had an option, I preferred smoking a joint to getting silly with alcohol.

This pain in my head was obviously a physical reaction to the stressful process of trying to create a sophisticated version of a mainstream film, so I went out to a shopping centre with Russell's bodyguard friend and bought a full sports kit. I got shoes, socks and a whole bunch of clothes that I would need for running. I had to do something about myself. By taking care of my body I would surely get better. Paracetamol and other pills didn't seem to lessen the pain. I talked to a few people in the supermarket pharmacies of LA, but as I wasn't signed up to any health plan they didn't want to talk to me.

The day of the read-through, I woke up early, put on my

new black sports kit, parked my car by the Greek Theater and dashed all the way up to the top of the Hollywood hills. Sweating and gasping for breath, I viewed the world from up there. The ocean was beautiful, as was the late January air, which had started cleaning my tobacco-clogged lungs. I was sure that everything was going to be fine – how could it not be? I went back, took a shower and started preparing for that afternoon's show.*

~

My hope, my vanity and my yearning for self-affirmation were all there as a team of black text, travelling together on a 110-page journey to my future. There, in the garden of Starbucks, I lit up a cigarette and waited for the tattooed guy who worked in the Kinko's across the street to print me fifteen copies. Like an anxious dad at the first day of school, I had handed him *Bad Father* with exact instructions on how it needed to be laid out. The LA hipster listened with bored indifference. He knew it all already. It was LA, after all, and he didn't need explanations about how to print a film script. He promptly pulled out a big box of paper, stuck my name on it and said, as if to calm me down, 'It will be ready in an hour and a half.'

My headache had subsided, so I could finally look at what Paul had come up with to finish off act three. While holding page ninety-one open with my left hand, I blew air on to my cup of odd-smelling Tazo chai tea. It was showtime and I needed a proper kick. My idea of moving from American coffee to Indian tea was all part, I thought, of my physical regeneration. That morning's tea was very sweet and, probably because of that, addictive. I have never doubted that in America, more

---

* Margarita: 'That day before your operation we had a Skype conversation entirely full of love. You told me that you had been getting a lot of headaches, but that in the morning you had been running up the hills with Tom. Your skin was luminous, your eyes were almost sparkling. I felt an intense love for you . . . and then look what happened. That was the last Skype of our old life.'

than in any other culture, they can package and sell you almost anything, from healthcare to Maccy D's, and the next day you'll be back yearning for more.

I looked around the café. I was surrounded by other people like me, who were following the American dream, and who, at some point, had started doing yoga and drinking green juices and Asian teas, and were now talking confidently about their next great film, or their next great TV series, which would bring them instant success.

In that land of opportunity, we would all find happiness or resolution, or at least confirmation of our own ego. Crucially, in that town, you learn that 'You Gotta Smile'. It's not such a bad thing, to smile at everyone. If you love them or hate them, just smile. This was the place where I could finally stop smoking and get healthy.

As I focused on the script and started reading, I did not just enter the fictional world of *Bad Father*, I started travelling through the last pages of my own life as I knew it. While trying to follow the dialogue between my precious characters, I must have got lost, or distracted, because I continuously had to stop and accept that I did not remember the sentence I had just read. My naps and healthy walks in the Hollywood hills had obviously not been enough to cure me of whatever I had.

It soon became clear that my brain was shifting my thoughts in directions beyond my control. As my mind wandered, I recognized that I had been forcing every part of my brain to come up with the best story turns for the third act, so it was perhaps not too surprising if something in my parking lot of ideas had short-circuited.

The fact that I had driven my car there, without any problems, meant there was no reason for me to be anxious. While drunks are not conscious of how badly they are driving, the worst thing that most stoners do is to drive their car very slowly. My brain was more stoned than drunk.

Gradually I realized that there was an Alien being forcing itself into my story, no longer allowing me to direct it or produce it myself.

This is not the point in the story where I started to lose my ability to read. Not yet at least. You have to be patient, and wait a while longer before we get to that scene. You'll recognize it when you get there, as there are many broken clocks that surround and change the perspective of the narrative. But my relationship with letters and strange exterior characters does begin to crackle at this moment.

As my short-term memory burned away in my brain, I forgot just about everything from that script. It took me the whole of that hour and a half to go through those twenty-five pages and the only thing that I understood was that Paul had not managed to finish the whole thing. There were about ten more pages still missing, the ones that would surprise the audience and give us the magic three endings, which I had really wanted to push through the narrative.

What had I been doing during that hour and a half? I did not find my cup of sweet tea anywhere – had I finished it? At what point did I stand up to throw it away?

~

When I walked into Russell's house with the fifteen printed copies of the script in my hands, everybody seemed excited at the prospect of doing some proper acting. As they all walked up to his room on the top floor, Paul and I sat down with him to lay out who was going to read which character. I saw a sticker that I had posted on the big box of paper, which reminded me to tell him about the missing ten pages. After just a minuscule pause, that for me felt endless, his mouth opened.

'You can't do a read-through of a story that isn't finished. Let's tell everybody that it's cancelled.'

I looked at Paul, smiled, pulled myself together, and in my calmest and most reassuring voice, said, 'Those last pages are just details. I read through the whole thing while waiting for the hipster to print them all, and the story is all there. Don't worry.'

Russell looked into my eyes as only he can, giving me full responsibility for what was about to happen, and said, 'OK. Let's do it,' then stood up and went to greet the other friends who had arrived.

Everybody had a role to read apart from me. I refused to participate, as I knew from my morning funny-tea breakfast that my eyes were strangely not working very well. I sat alone in front of the whole cast, which made me feel like a king, enjoying a private performance. When, at the halfway point of the script, Tom called for a ten-minute break, Russell picked up a cigarette and went out to the terrace, expecting me to join him. The mere movements of the various bodies walking past me were making me feel slightly off balance, as if I were on a boat in the middle of a storm, so I stayed sitting in my chair.

Everyone, including Russell and Nik, looked happy. They had laughed and seemed surprised. The reaction during the second half of the read-through was even better. I felt their energy, but somehow I could not quite follow the text. It was as if this crew of lovely people was talking to me in a foreign language, without noticing that my only contribution was a continuous smile and a head movement. Since I now knew that the story worked, I didn't care. I felt fine.

Everybody congratulated Paul and me for a good job, and started preparing for that evening's show. For the next three nights, Russell and Nik had hired a crew to film the narrative part of their *Happiness* documentary. (Did I tell you about this documentary already? My short-term memory really seems to have disappeared, and is now travelling, together with my reading, in a wormhole in my head. But of all the things that I can repeat, I guess *Happiness* is not the worst.)

It was a very important story for Russell, as it documented his entrance into the world of superstars, and his emotional reaction to it. The more famous he was, the more he realized that the whole game was just a distraction from reality. While contributing to a global addiction to superstars, he needed to find a way of narrating his own critique of it. As a recovering addict, he knew that what you think you love and need is often a barrier to real happiness, whatever that might be.

Meanwhile my headache was reasserting itself and I was becoming overwhelmed by pain. I lay down on a couch by the door, and waited for an old friend of mine from Oberlin College (a liberal arts school in Ohio, where we had both spent the early 1990s) to come and pick me up. Like me, Kenneth Francis had been a bass player in various college bands and I was sure that he would help me find a doctor who could sort out my headaches. Kenneth arrived and away we went. I was still buzzing from what I thought was my headache and I could hardly communicate with my old pal. He took me to several different clinics, but I was told they had no space for me there. As soon as they discovered that I did not have any health insurance, they became uninterested in my problems.

As a second, a third, and a fourth rejection followed, my perception of the world started becoming fainter and fainter, and my friend, realizing that he could no longer communicate with me, felt lost. His words stopped having a meaning for me. It was not particularly stressful. It was just sound, with no information. A rhythm with no shape.

As the moon had risen and the evening traffic had subsided, Kenneth, extremely anxious by now, picked up his phone. 'Hey, Dad. I have an old friend of mine from Oberlin here with me, and he seems to be losing . . . he no longer seems able to answer, or maybe even hear my questions. He has a really bad headache . . . and he doesn't have any health insurance.' After a long pause, 'It's ten-thirty here in LA.' Another brief pause. 'The nearest one is the Kaiser Permanente down Sunset, not far . . . Thanks, Dad, I'll find the ER there.'

As Kenneth stopped his car on a completely empty street, he told me something that I could not understand, but the movement of his arm indicated that I should open my door and step out. As he bent down, closed my door and drove off, I saw that I was near the entrance to a hospital. I followed the slow movement of his car, as it searched for a parking spot. The headache had almost subsided, or rather, had reached such overwhelming power that I could no longer recognize it as pain.

I sat down on the floor, a bit dizzy and weak. I heard no cars and no people; I just saw the bright light of the doors of the ER, heard the humming of the gigantic air-conditioning units, and wondered what film it reminded me of. It wasn't a horror film, even though it was something of that genre. It also definitely wasn't a comedy or a romance. Was I in a real location? Or a set? Was I in reality?

Kenneth arrived, picked me up from the floor and accompanied me into the ER, where, after being helped to fill in the paperwork, I was accepted and taken in. Someone must have told him that he could go home and not worry, because they were going to take good care of me. At the time, I had no way of imagining the Alien attack and simply assumed that a doctor would appear; she would give me a proper painkiller, tell me to get a good sleep there in the ER, and that would be it.

How could I possibly have anticipated that the Aliens would arrive in our biosphere and choose me, out of all the people of the world running around and excited to meet them? I was too tired and weak, so I allowed those Alien forces that had been trying to take over my head, to procreate as they wanted.

This is what happened in my brain as I passed out in the ER of that hospital.

Aliens? What? I had never planned for my story to incorporate those kinds of characters. While I have appreciated *Alien*, *Aliens* and particularly *Alien 3*, I am definitely not going to cast such creatures in my first Hollywood film. No. Ouch . . .

pain, a lot of pain in my head . . . That was undeniably an attack. A proper exhibition of violence and hate. What have I done to deserve this?

It could not . . . Ouch . . . what the hell? Could it be because of that gap? Those open ten pages that weren't finished? Did someone, or better, something, enter into my story that way? Is it, like everyone in this town, desperately in need of affirmation? Of fame? HHHHaaaa . . . Why *my* head? No. Someone from the read-through would have made me notice that Paul or I had, by mistake, put one of those characters into a scene of the story.

Come on! *Bad Father* is a romantic comedy, and it has been created to make you laugh and maybe even cry a little, but I can't really see the sense of an action scene in the third act. Yes, the more Big Boom Bang there is in a Hollywood film, the more money they make. They have proved on various occasions that with enough money you can resolve almost everything. Here, they certainly do have the money. What is . . . aaAhhh . . . maybe I simply have to change the narrative and hire a special effects team, who can make the Aliens' spaceship, or whatever they arrived in, piss off back to their own shitty reality.

You Alien people . . . beings . . . you seem to have an even bigger ego problem than my friend Russell. You are continuously interrupting me . . . I am talking about you . . . yes, I am, and yes . . . there's no way you'll become the most important characters of my life. You fucking egomaniac bastards. I had projects . . . I was writing important stories that were going to revolutionize cinematic history . . . Ouch . . .! Fuck off!!

They couldn't have been living here, in my reality. Maybe they have been frozen somewhere in the North Pole, and now, due to global warming, have decided to attack, of all things, my cheating priest. Look. Whoever you are. Have you seen *Take Him to the Greek*? Russell can definitely carry a film himself, we really don't need . . . Ouchhh . . . Fuck! . . . I am trying to say something important here, and you Alien dudes seem to have a very heightened sense of self-importance. Why do you want to make me pay for it? It really hurts!

AAAAhh! What happens if, at this stage, and considering what is now happening to the third act of the script, I play my trump card? Jack, I know you didn't want the voice of God in this story, but as we hadn't talked about the possible arrival of Aliens . . . I am going to override your wish, and bring him in. That is, if you, God, want to? I assume you don't have a Holly-spirit type agent I have to talk to?

Or are you actually pissed off because I didn't fight your corner vigorously enough in the first stage of development? Come on! You are the Almighty, the all-forgiving. Give me a break. I was just trying to learn the rules of this new American economy. Cross my fingers and . . . well, I promise you that in the next film, where I will have more power and control of the narrative, I will definitely give you an important role. Ouchhh . . . I'll give you a . . . obviously, I'll make you the main character . . . I am losing this war. The film is going to be shit!

And . . . And . . . Am I actually dying? Is this what is happening? I need help. Help me.

Note to Alex: To help my memory go back in time, remember to read me something by Italo Calvino . . . as he has always been helpful for my more historical tales.

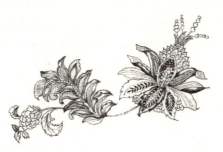

4

Anarchism Through Comedy

London, 1999–2002

Alex has recently read me an article about the 'Medical liability crisis for safety net hospitals', which, in its extremely oblique way, defines my situation in LA; nevertheless, I think of it rather as the tale of a human being who stupidly walked into the United States of America without health insurance, and I will leave my political commentary on the hidden meanings behind that subject till a bit later.

Dr Vogel told me he had no doubt that I would have died in

one of those macabre low-income safety nets, so I should certainly give credit to my comedian friend, Russell Brand, as I feel that somewhere on that evening he saved my life. The fact that neither Russell nor I have been particularly concerned about the details of him saving my life, is due to a series of rather comedic incidents that took place in a dim and distant past.

In order to elucidate our man-to-man relationship, I will have to, again, bring you back in time. It will be something like 'thirteen years before' . . . at the turn of the century.

~

This chapter starts right there in 1999, as Russell, shortly after we had met, convinced me to help make him, and his presence in the world of media, ubiquitous.

I had never met a person whose principal aim in life was to be recognized as a silhouette. There are very few characters whom you can recognize as a cut-up piece of black paper. The first that come to my mind are Walt Disney's Mickey Mouse or Goofy, but standing there, looking at Russell's image reflected on the mirror of his bathroom in his stinky shared flat (I think it was near Oval station) which reeked of hair gel and hairspray, he showed me his favourite silhouettes of Groucho Marx with his moustache and cigar, and Charlie Chaplin with his hat and stick. Somehow this justified why his hair looked the way it did – somewhere between a fashion show and a mental hospital.

As an Italian in America, I was used to being seen as a man who took care of his attire, and throughout my life I have enjoyed experimenting with my hair, beard and mustachio, but that was my first 'Branded' lesson about the importance of marketing yourself by being immediately recognizable.

I won't get into Jungian discussions of Russell and myself playing with reality and wanting to use media to light up the shadows (at least not yet), but I am sure that somewhere in this chapter, you might ask yourself about the psychology of our characters and which of us is more insane. (Or 'Who's the more foolish, the fool or the fool who follows him?', as Obi-Wan Kenobi would say.)

You'll soon understand that one of my great talents, and a recurring theme in my life, has been to get myself into seemingly impossible situations. After all, I have managed to get to Chapter Four relatively unscathed, which – ask Alex – was no easy task.

Note to Alex: I really do mean unscathed, not unshaved, although that is also true.

I am going to love writing this chapter, because I have realized that I have a much easier time recalling my more ancient history. I am forty-one years old right now, and while writing about the events that happened in my twenties, I am not confronted with my short-term memory. After having worked intensively on remembering all the details of my recent drama, it feels good to take out that edge, and work with Alex on the parts of this tale that I actually do remember.

~

London, it was 1999 (I said that a few times already, right?), and let's start this chapter with a woman. Yes, I was trying to help my friend Emily, who had brought me into this film-making industry just a few years before, to narrate *A Brief History of Cuba in D Minor*, a twenty-three-minute musical. This seemingly foolish venture was made possible by the success of our first film, where we had flipped on its head Danish film director Lars von Trier's Dogme movement with humour and music. That film school 'documentary' had been sold in several different countries, and had even received a 'Best Student Film in the World' award. So, yes, the world was our oyster.

Emily and I set the rules of our documentary game by playing with our common interest in postmodern philosophy and in particular the question of who decides what is the history that we want to remember, and how the media is continuously shaping the past for its own needs.

Casting such an unusual 'documentary' was a challenge. For most actors this low-budget film-school project must have seemed either ridiculous or mad – or truly visionary. At that moment, Russell Brand walked into my life. He arrived at the casting accompanied by four cans of beer and a beautiful Spanish woman. Our composer had managed to create a score that, following Emily's vision, sounded like a 1960s American musical, performed in a Cuban theatre. Russell's voice was good, as was his version of a Cuban-American accent, and as he walked out of the room, I immediately went to Emily and told her that I had no doubt we had to cast him. I found that there was something extremely charming about that man.

So a few weeks later, Amanda (the Spanish woman), his cans of beer and a joint, accompanied Russell into the NFTS studio outside London to record his character's music score, to which he would later have to dance. Russell sang his parts professionally, even if he was a bit drunk, and we were all satisfied.

On the morning of the shoot, as I walked around the empty stage, the sensation was thrilling. In a few hours, I knew that room would be completely filled up and I would be responsible for this huge production. But then, while Emily and I were outside smoking a cigarette and talking through the technical details of the green screen, we were interrupted by a phone call. On the other end, I heard Russell's shy voice. He told me that he had put his back out and that he could neither dance nor stand on his feet.

I put down the phone, told Emily about our new crisis, and after a few minutes of looking comically bewildered at each other, she started singing me a song from *Singing in the Rain*. The one that goes 'Good Morning, Good Morning . . .' and we had a solution to our seemingly impossible problem. When our dance coach arrived on set, I took him for a walk, and brought him back half an hour later wearing the clothes of Russell's character, which fortunately, with only a few stitches, fitted him perfectly.

Six months afterwards, when Emily and I were finishing the post-production of *A Brief History of Cuba*, Russell came back into the studio and told me that he had just auditioned for an

MTV show and was sure he was going to become their new presenter. It seemed like a great gig, which would get him off his English teaching job and on to a proper performing employ-ment that would pay him a considerable amount of money, but he did not seem satisfied. He had not even been confirmed or hired, and he was already talking about wanting more. He seemed convinced that together, he and I could do much better than anything the MTV creative team had come up with. I liked him and his cockiness and was curious to see what he could do.

I organized a shoot with him, and I brought Emily with me both as spiritual support and as camerawoman. Russell and I had met a few days before and he laid out a plan, where he would attempt to prove that he could eliminate money from all human transactions. That morning, he drank three shots of whisky and a bottle of beer, and as we started moving around Camden Market, he began by trying to trade a romantic song for a cup of coffee. The song was funny enough that the bartender gave him his coffee, and followed Russell's dance of success with a wry smile.

As Russell circulated all day, trading kisses and dances for everything possible on the market, like socks, pencils, bread and carrots, I noticed that the people we encountered found him at the same time strange and compelling. By the end of the day, tired and physically exhausted, we hopped on a bus, where Russell even managed to convince a conductor to swap a ride for a flower. It worked. We actually got a happy ending for our short story.

That evening, on our way home, Russell and I looked at each other and realized that by working together, 'The revolution *will* be televised', and Russell Brand would be presenting it. Within a week we set up our first production company, and called it Vanity Projects. Our aim was humble. Television, radio, films, we were going to use whatever came our way in order to bring the enlightening power of comedy to the masses.

While doing the rounds to find Russell a new agent, I noticed that he was easily bored by the endless corporate chatter and so used those occasions to show off. I had never seen a person behave like that, but I guess that now that he was presenting a night-time show for MTV he had his choice, and could control the mood of a room and test the character of those people.

When talking to John, the director of the John Noel agency, Russell picked up a little plastic ball of the globe that was lying on his desk, sat upside down on a couch, and with his feet up in the air started juggling it against the wall. John was not fazed by this performance and as we left his office gave Russell that little globe to keep. Russell walked out on to the street yelling, 'I am the king of the world! I am king of the world!', quoting Leonardo DiCaprio (in the scene from his famous film where he stands on top of a big boat that predictably, in the middle of the second act, has to sink).

We hopped on a very crowded Tube, where Russell's energy could not be mitigated. He spotted a beautiful, big-breasted girl standing amongst the various other squeezed bodies reading their newspapers, held his globe up and got her attention. In his limited Spanish, he tried to seduce her through the crowd. I was looking at this operation with absolute certainty that the only result would be a few people smiling at his sad pick-up attempt. Before we got off the Tube he disappeared, and while I was walking up the stairs, smiling to myself, he resurfaced next to me with a piece of paper in his hand and a big-ass smile on his face, and said, 'I'll see her tomorrow night!'

What bonded us from the beginning was the awareness that we were a natural odd couple. We each had clear aims and while understanding that my grooves inspired his seemingly endless improvisations, we became more excited by where our partnership was going to take us. To Russell's anti-conformist look and attitude, I put the language and sharpness of an over-educated politician. With his silhouettes in his mind, Russell knew better than I did how the media is all about images and so we played with every part of it.

We were two different character roles with a shared excitement – which was most clearly exemplified by our strange choices of fashion and hairstyle. We made friends with all the new East End artisans and Russell, who was now earning good money, started wearing suits, created in a little shop where they used only recycled fabrics to create a kind of postmodern fashion style. He had a few proper business suits where the fabric of the arms had been cut halfway and substituted with similarly coloured sections from sports jackets. Emily had already introduced me to her East End hairdressers who were experimenting with strong colours and shapes, and I (still with little money) gave them free range to try out different styles on my head. One of the best haircuts I ever had the pleasure of receiving was black, straight hair, cut on a slant from left to right (I would love to show that to Dr Vogel at some point). Many of our new friends and collaborators were Italians, who worked with Japanese or Brits, who were inspired by Germans, and it was clear for us that we were standing on the edge of an inevitable postmodernity, which we were helping to create.

I knew two girls in London who never took drugs. They were the exception to the rule, though; everybody around me went out and freely consumed drugs of almost every type. There were plenty of clubs where every single person was either on acid or somehow tripping. I did not consider smoking joints as being a drug, because in my life that was as common as drinking beer. It even cost less than drinking beer.

A few years before, after finishing my Cambridge postgraduate degree, I had moved directly to London, where alcohol was from the very start a fundamental part of my life. While during the day I tried to make my degree work for me and wrote articles for economy trade magazines, at night I was a bartender, mixing cocktails in a dodgy place in Brixton, where criminals from South London loved to drink my fancy shakes and the security man drove a Rolls-Royce.

I was constantly trying to sneak some radicalism into my

finance or banking articles, something that could give that job a meaning. In fact (my brain really does work better when I go back in time), I remember that the only article I was really proud of was called 'Do Banks Dream of Electric Sheep?' quoting ironically the *Blade Runner* future created by Philip K. Dick. But like most of my Cambridge professors, the bankers financing the magazines had very little feeling for comedy or irony, and that's probably why my cocktails remained my primary source of income.

Emily would come to the bar in the afternoons and, while I was serving drinks or cleaning the various bottles of vodka, we bounced ideas about, and thought of interesting ways of narrating the truth with films. The fact that, after closing hours, the local gangster would stand by the bar drinking whisky and playing with his Stanley knife, and would ask me how films are created, made me realize that being a film maker could give you power. As the narrator of the stories, you were creating the truth that you wanted the world to believe. It was a new language for me, which neither photographs nor newspaper articles could express. My apologies for this diversion, but now you know to attribute my entry into this industry in part to being good at mixing cocktails for gangsters.

Russell eventually chose the most powerful and posh agency in town, which represented the biggest stars. Within a few weeks, we had developed five different TV comedy series which, with the help of his new agent, we were going to take to the UK channels to get commissioned. I had heard that getting one show commissioned could take quite a while, but we were sure that with five in our hands, at least one would *certainly* break through.

Before doing that, we had to take a little trip to Edinburgh for the comedy fringe festival, where Russell was going to spice up his presentation of some new young comedians with a few of his latest jokes. Russell had always been madly self-aware of his own character and created all his comedy on the basis of his own life, so much so that many of his daily decisions were driven by their potential to become part of his show.

Shortly after his rather unique presentation, he disappeared. After a few hours' talking with some TV commissioners, I started getting worried. Russell would have told me if he had gone anywhere. I asked the various men working in security if they had seen a tall, oddly clad man passing by. 'Yes,' said one of them and directed me to the police, who told me that Russell had been brought into the A & E of Edinburgh's biggest hospital an hour earlier.

I found him lying down in his hospital bed, trying to make the policemen laugh. He saw me arrive and smiled like a wicked boy who was aware of having done something wrong. He told me that two of the comedy club's security guards had not liked his general attitude, and somehow ended up throwing him out of the club through a glass door. I saw that his right leg had been cut quite badly and told him, 'Now you're going to tell me how you're going to make this into your next piece of comedy.'

The week after, on the basis of an eight-minute 'taster' that we had shot with Emily and some contacts of his new agent, we started having meetings with various TV stations around town. We thought we had prepared our pitch quite well and, after the necessary office small talk, we would present them with our little show. We would turn on a CD, with music and Russell's voice singing, and I would pull out a stack of white pages with single words on them, which Russell would throw away one by one, in the style of Bob Dylan in the video of 'Subterranean Homesick Blues'. We surprised them and gave them all the material they could want and even managed to make the whole experience quite cool. What else could they wish for?

The biggest one, Channel 4, liked the presentation and our attitude. They offered us the possibility of making a thirty-minute episode of one of our projects for them, and if they liked what they saw, maybe we could talk again. Perhaps we were a bit cocky, but we were not convinced by that deal, and so kept on looking around.

A young man in a new TV station had called me a few times and seemed very eager to meet us. We arrived on time in their gigantic modern building and after waiting for twenty minutes Russell started getting itchy. Holding him down after having drunk five espressos and a shot of alcohol was understandably difficult. When finally, forty-five minutes late, the assistant to the head of the channel came down to pick us up, Russell was already in his own, alternative reality. He walked about with a huge emergency fire extinguisher in his arms, pointing it at everyone as we passed by. He had decided it was a present for the people in our meeting who had made us wait so long.

That was not all, for as soon as we heard that the top boss was not even going to appear at the meeting, Russell smiled, pulled down his trousers and sat down with his naked butt, saying cheerfully, 'Let's start, then!'

I was charmed by Russell's seemingly crazy antics. In fact, I had the sensation that the entrance of such an eccentric character into those corporate agencies was leaving a memorable trail. They all needed to show the world, and their financiers, that they were new, brave and edgy. A few days later, I received a phone call from the TV station, telling me that they were considering giving us a series of ten half-hour comedies. Even if the budget they were offering for each episode was quite small, we could definitely do something with it. We had our own TV show!

Now that we had a television channel in hand, we went in search of a bigger production company that could embrace us and help us to put together the paperwork and finance needed for us to start rolling the camera. In the end we chose Vera, where some of our favourite political satire shows had been created. The boss was a lovely, warm man with buckets of experience, and from the first time we walked into their offices we had the sensation that they shared our vision, in which political engagement, entertainment and humour had to live together.

With their help we laboriously negotiated a deal for the ten-part show with that new, upcoming TV station. Finally, I could get out of bartending and start paying rent from my own creative endeavours. Most importantly we were in a position to experiment and learn the tools of the trade. We were racing to the top, and could physically sense how the world was being attracted towards us.

What made me very excited about all the projects we had in development was that we were using a Hi-Lo production method. We were going to show the TV audience that the proletariat is not dumb and that the posh people don't have to live with a stick up their asses. We could appreciate 'Art' together with humour, and bring them to bond with each other, rather than continuously fight.

We had found the channel, the production company, some money and some new friends in the cool East End, so everything was looking rosy. It was our dream come true. How could it not succeed?

~

Russell and I lived very close to each other, near Hackney Road in East London, and so every morning I would walk down from my apartment in a council estate, which I shared with two sweet but stinky Polish boys, who cleaned the kitchen in a restaurant near Bank Tube station, and a Spanish couple who were waiters in a tapas restaurant. I would pick up a copy of the *Guardian* and a pack of rolling tobacco and turn into Russell's street, where I would usually find an Addison Lee minicab waiting downstairs for us. He would leave the front door open for me, as he was always in the bathroom getting ready.

I have met very few men who take so much time doing their hair, but now that he was on television I guess it was excused. Through his presenter job at MTV he was becoming a public character, a person who journalists had started to keep an eye on. I don't think that the private taxi was supposed to be used outside of his work for MTV, but I didn't have a problem with it. After all, it was a good sign that our lives were moving in the right direction.

Morning traffic from the east side of London is terrible and we would surely have arrived in town much faster on the underground. Even when we left the house late, Russell would insist that the driver stop by the corner shop where he would pick up his day's papers – the *Sun*, the *Mirror* and the *Telegraph* – and I accepted it all, as it was my morning's British Reality class for beginners. This lesson had nothing to do with my presumptuous Cambridge professors – this was what the majority of British people read every morning, and so, how life and politics were interpreted. My copy of the *Guardian* would almost always end up lying unopened next to me, as Russell would read me the most angry and homophobic articles of the *Sun*. It was a sincerely complex world for me. Everybody in this country simply accepted the fact that this newspaper, the most popular paper in the country, always had a half-naked woman looking at you from page three.

In my more academic, American brain I thought about the cultural implications of this chauvinist tradition, but then I had to stop. I had almost forgotten that where I grew up, in Italy, all the mainstream television shows opened with a team of semi-naked women jiggling their breasts and smiling.

I often talked with Russell about the parallels between the British and Italian chauvinist attitude, but while we agreed politically, there was a fundamental difference between our approach. Call it culture, call it class, call it whatever you want, but Russell was a sexist. Conscious and self-critical, maybe, but he could not take his eyes off those big breasts.

Every morning, as we arrived in the large open-plan office at Vera, the company that was executive producing our show, Russell would start playing his favourite game. Keeping his attention while we were in that office was more than difficult for me. It was like putting a five-year-old boy in a children's wonderland full of toys and chocolate and expecting him to pay attention to the details of a timeline for one of our ten episodes. In this case it really wasn't a problem of chauvinism; it was the women working there who forced the situation with continuous little smiles and laughs. While we were sitting there at our desk, his head was in a constant callisthenic exercise of left to right and back again.

One particular morning, I set Russell down next to our work table in the corner of the office and tried to get his attention, but since his eyes were clearly elsewhere, I decided to take him out for coffee in one of the many gay bars in Old Compton Street. I needed his full attention. I had spent the whole night working and thought that I had cracked the structure that would allow us to make this ten half-hour series fun, exciting and constantly surprising.

As I lit a cigarette and started pitching him the idea, he looked at the people walking by and suddenly interrupted me with his hand, signalling a one-minute break. He walked briskly across the road and started chatting with one of his homeless friends. They disappeared in a corner alleyway, leaving me with a half-thought on my tongue and a gay bartender asking me if everything was fine. I told him, 'No. It is not fine. Not fine at all.'

After an endless amount of time Russell reappeared. This time around he looked different, and he spoke differently. He was looking at me lackadaisically, responding to my complaints with a simple smile. Yes, he had met his lover. He had a new story with a woman who neither had big breasts, nor a beautiful face; she was foreign and common, scary and annoying – her name was Heroine.

Alex has mistakenly spelled 'heroin' here as 'Heroine', but in a way, that is correct, too.

This new love for heroin became my worst enemy. All excuses, all failures, all confusions were packed into the 'drugbrella'.

This was Russell's word for when he was under the influence of hard drugs, his excuse always being, 'I was underneath my drugbrella.' I now had to share a space in that bloody drugbrella and depend on the whims of a comedian and his lover, Heroine.

He put a lot of effort into making comedy out of his addiction, but it was clear that this hero of his was distracting even his natural comedy rhythms. I don't know which was worse, to see my company slowly collapse, or to live with a friend whose life and character were dependent on his quick-witted reaction time and who had noticeably started to lose his beats and comedy.

To make my life just a bit more complicated, as soon as the TV commissioners signed the contract with Vera we had both moved to bigger and nicer houses, which raised my financial stakes considerably. While I shared a two-floor apartment with Adrian Muys, the younger brother of my best friend from college, who was a big, athletic American boy and had a sensible job working as an investment banker in the City, Russell got himself a big flat right next to a bar where I used to work, and in which all the best drug dealers loved to hang out.

The only positive part of this bloody drama was that Russell hated the idea of being pricked with needles in his arms or anywhere else. The other option, for more squeamish heroin consumers, is what is commonly called 'chasing the dragon' – where a person cuts a piece of tinfoil and puts some heroin on it, heats it underneath with a cigarette lighter, and then inhales the resulting smoke through a tube of rolled-up foil.

Whenever I saw Russell with a piece of tinfoil in his bag or in his pocket, my emotions would start to shake. It was just tinfoil. Like a lonely, jealous wife throwing the good dinner plates on to a wall to hear them crash, I hid or threw away every type of tinfoil that I found. I had seen *Drugstore Cowboy* and read enough books to know that the risk factor of this situation was extremely high. Just a few months before, we would spend entire evenings working through various ideas and hopes; now none of this interested him. The common response was, 'Yeah, great . . . Yeah . . .' One of the sharpest and quickest brains I had ever met was there swimming with his friend heroin in their drugbrella and asking me to please give them back their tinfoil.

From the beginning of our work with Vera, the whole staff liked us exactly because we were young, energetic, a bit wild, brought excitement into their life and had good politics. Russell had presented the new name of our show to the whole office; it was going to be called IWATTIRTWWHCWTE. He insisted that it was going to be called that and everyone should try to use that name. The full version went as follows: 'It Was At This Time I Realized That What We Had Created Was Truly Evil.'

Sadly I hadn't yet met Margarita, my psychiatrist wife, as I would have very much liked to hear her opinion of our new name, and what the hell was happening in our brains when we chose it.

A few months later, I had to walk into the office of our executive producer with a very different kind of proposition. From the very beginning we had embraced him as our revolutionary father figure, who had endless belief in us, so I was a bit sad to have to tell him about . . . well, drugbrella. I tried my best, and presented him with the new version of our show like this: 'In the first episodes of our series . . . hold on to something sturdy . . . we will film Russell kicking his addiction to heroin . . . and while we shoot the other episodes we will regularly come back to his addiction and relationship with heroin all the way to the tenth episode, where we'll see him starting a new life, clean of this drug.'

My explanation was that if anything could force Russell to give up his comfortable place in drugbrella, it would be the reality that, by publicly kicking the habit, the doors to fame would open for him. This show would break all the rules and surprise everyone. After this long-winded presentation, I took a pause. Our Exec was not looking me in the eye and I had a very bad premonition. The entrance of our unglamorous 'Heroine' into the show was not what he had signed up for. For the first time ever, he looked sincerely worried.

A few days later, our cameraman Matt Morgan, whom Russell had met in his MTV show, his girlfriend and I went to Russell's house and filmed him while taking his 'last dose of heroin'. It was shot well and we knew we were doing the right thing. Matt's camera followed Russell and me afterwards hugging and celebrating The End, but somehow it all seemed too easy. Could it have been because he looked too joyful, there in his drug-brella? I walked away from his house with some doubts, which the next morning were quickly confirmed, as I passed by the kitchen to get him up and saw a bit of tinfoil lying on the middle of the table. It was clearly going to be much more difficult than I expected.

I had invested too much of my soul in this and I wasn't going to get knocked down by that drug. So, after having considered all the various options, we found what we believed was . . . the cure. We were going to make our ten-part series on a bus! Yes, we would hire a large camper van and physically take Russell out of London, as far away from his dealers as geograph-ically possible. We had set up encounters with various characters throughout Great Britain, who could generate inter-esting comedy. If Russell didn't have his dealers, he could not get drugs, and we could thus heal him and make our TV show.

Our first stop was in a museum of art by the sea. Russell was going to pass by the port, pick up some fresh fish, and then nail it on a frame and take it to the director of the art museum, asking her to please hang it among their other art pieces.

It was a time when Damien Hirst was greatly appreciated for showing us the bodies of various animals preserved in formal-dehyde and sometimes dissected for our artistic . . . excitement? And so, this somehow legitimized the first stop of our trip.

I don't remember exactly why, but Russell had somehow convinced me that at the end of the shoot we absolutely had to set our camper van on fire and watch it blow up. Since I don't like the word 'No' while I am working, I came up with the idea of buying an old beat-up camper van, which we could repaint in different ways as each episode finished. Financially it was possible, but somehow, as Vera started to lose faith in my dreamy presentations, I found myself in front of a big, rented, well-kept camper van, which did look like a more pragmatic way to travel.

That morning Russell, Matt Morgan, our director, our new executive producer and I were all going to leave together in our hired camper van. Yes, from the moment that the issue of heroin had entered into our story, Vera had introduced one of their execs to keep an eye on us. We had galvanized participation by all the Vera staff for our departure and various office girls had made us sandwiches and bought us soft drinks. It felt like a group of pilots attempting the first transoceanic flight.

As I had pitched it to Vera's Exec, our project seemed like the story of Charles Lindbergh's first solo flight across the Atlantic Ocean, which propelled him into global fame. Nevertheless, as we were getting closer to our own departure, I did start thinking of the two French pilots who had attempted the flight the other way around just a few weeks before and had disappeared, never to be found.

As Matt and I put our bags in the camper van, we smiled. It was a properly crazy idea. I called Russell to make sure that he was arriving, a bit worried that he had packed his bag properly – without hidden stashes in his socks or pockets. He arrived with a bottle of whisky in his hand and another for us. We walked into this very posh camper van and while he was drinking his whisky-juice mix, decided that we had everything and it was time to depart.

Russell walked outside, looked at our little audience of girls from the office, then found that there were steps on the back of the camper, so he climbed up to the roof. He stood up there looking down and seemed truly happy. We smiled at him as the Vera producer quickly told him that he had to get down immediately, as we were not covered for such things.

I guess there are moments in everyone's life that become

history, which will never be erased from your mind. This twinkle in reality took the top prize. From that moment on, it would remain forever in my head as the 'Van Roof' moment. Yes, because after about half an hour of us all trying to tell Russell to stop being an idiot and get down, the Vera producer pulled out his mobile phone to call the execs and cancel the trip.

I told him to hold his horses and climbed up to the roof to join Russell, who at this point was manic. I sat next to him, touched his hands and asked him what was wrong. Like a little child who has had his favourite toy taken away, he simply said, 'I want to be on this roof, why can't I be on this roof? Just let me go a little, really slowly. I want to be on this roof.' We looked each other in the eye and then we saw that the producer was already on the phone with the execs and cancelling it all. Russell saw my tears as they slipped down my face, and hugged me.

We climbed down, picked up our luggage from the camper van and walked away with Matt, leaving all the girls standing there completely bemused. We sat down in the first pub we found, to cool down and talk about what had just happened. Russell was now fully present, and was surprised himself at what had taken place. He understood why he'd done it, and was now facing the implications of his actions. What did this mean for our project?

In that moment Matt decided to put 'Van Roof' into our common lexicon, as a piece of text that we would all recognize, so that any time that Russell got really out of control, those two words would be spoken and would trigger him back to reality. We laughed and slowly made our way back to the office, where I was certain that I would have to take full responsibility for what had just taken place, and perhaps, even give the execs an explanation.

Back at the office, all the bosses were being briefed by their line producer on the events that had taken place. I was the next one in line and I didn't have many answers or explanations prepared for them. As I walked into the room with my tail between my legs, they immediately started telling me that I should never have climbed on top of the van with Russell.

I sat down, breathed in and looked at them incredulously. They were talking about that slight infringement of the rules when in fact a much, much bigger problem was in front of us. I was responsible for the event, but as the whole production was based on Russell's talent, and his very capacity for making comedy was now undermined by his use of drugs, we had a whole set of other, much larger, problems to tackle.

I spent the next week in bed, trying to sleep my sorrows away, and occasionally I would sit in the kitchen, smoke a cigarette and try to come up with some other creative production options that could magically deal with my problem. Russell and Matt also tried to throw some of their new ideas my way, but I realized that none of them would help us to resolve our underlying issue. On a cold summer day, I walked into Vera's office and sat down with both the bosses, and I told them that in light of Russell's situation, I could no longer produce the show. I stepped down.

After I finally signed off all those paper trails, I walked down to Oxford Street, where the rain had now started drizzling. The rhythm of London was just the same as ever. People were running, crossing with their umbrellas like a Formula One race, while I took that very public shower at a slow pace, conscious that someone had to take responsibility for what had happened. I walked from the centre of London, all the way to the East End, through a continuous shift between drizzle and rain, while contemplating where I would end up now.

When I arrived at Russell's, I told him about my meeting with the bosses and how I was now going to pack my bags and get someone else to take my room in my lovely flat. I knew that he felt guilty, and sad, and that we did not have much to talk about . . . apart from the fact that I should take off my clothes and get dry. I put on some of his ridiculous sports clothes, we hugged and said goodbye.

I boxed up all my belongings, parked them at a friend's flat and got on a plane back to Milan, then to Berlin, then to Paris, then to Rome. I guess I needed to find myself a job as far away as possible from any drugbrellas.

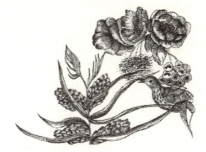

5

Hollywood and My Health

Los Angeles, 2011

As the car was pulling into our closed-off neighbourhood in Los Feliz, I looked up at the palm trees that continued up the hill, and nothing had really changed. I had only been away from that house for a week and it felt as if a year had passed. Had my time in the hospital just been a trick, or do I really have to find a way of telling my sun about Daddy's trip to the moon?

Note to Alex: I meant my 'son', of course, but I like the idea of Miro being my 'sun', so don't change it.

Would the battle against the Aliens be too intense for a three-year-old? At what age can I show him *Star Wars*, or my MRI for that matter?

As I walked into the house, I sensed an energy that surprised me; it all felt overwhelmingly normal and familiar. While my sister Bianca was stirring a pot in the kitchen, my mother Marianella was sitting outside reading a book. A light breeze floated through the windows as Margarita put her hand on my arm and took me around all the reorganized spaces, as if I were a tourist. Right behind the kitchen there was a little room, which had previously been used by the entourage to watch TV. I stepped in and there, kneeling down on a beige carpet, holding a train in his hand and buzzing the rhythm of *chuff, chuff,* I saw my boy, Miro. I hugged him and held him in my arms, and as his eyes rested on the left side of my head, he said, 'Do you have a boo-boo here?'

'Yes, but now I'm OK,' I told him.

He tried to touch it and kiss it, as we do with his boo-boos, but I was a bit scared by his quick hand movements and told him very quietly, 'Be really, really careful.'

Miro took my hand and proudly showed me the entire house, with a television hanging on the wall of every room and all of the toys that he had received for his birthday: the big train, his cuddly bear and his elephant were all sleeping calmly on his bed. He seemed really happy to see me. Who knows what had been going through his head the last few days? How could a three-year-old boy process all the emotions and fears that had been surrounding him? Now that his whole family was together, I guess he finally felt safe.

All of them looked settled, as if they had always been living there. I put on one of the big woolly hats that Nik had given me, in order not to scare anyone with my scars, and I joined

Miro's game with his trains, where he started answering me in a mixture of languages.

Since he was born, I have always spoken to him in English and have insisted on doing so, even if he only ever replied to me in Italian. He heard me speak Italian with his mum, and he had no problem with me flipping to a different language while talking to him, effortlessly following the stories of *Dr Seuss* and *Thomas the Tank Engine* that I read to him in bed.

This was the first time that I had ever heard him using English words, and while some of them must have come into his vocabulary from the cartoons that he had been watching here in America, he had some others with an unusual tone. I laughed out loud when I realized that at age three, my son had started learning some proper London cockney. Russell's bodyguard friend had been the one who had been playing with him the most. While my family was living through some very tense days, that delightful giant of a man had been there, playing with my boy.

While trying to come to terms with the concept of being ill, I found myself looking for a language that would allow me to communicate that terrible name, which carries with it such an awful historical stigma – *cancer*. I have never been interested in joining social clubs like the masons and I certainly did not want to be part of this exclusive oncology members' 'family', as I knew that once you are in, you never get out.

I had a cut in my head, so what? That didn't really mean anything, aside from the fact that I had to find a shop in LA that made cool hats. There was no way that I was going to be knocked down by words that I didn't even understand.

This was no doubt a self-defence mechanism, but to this day, when those oncological words appear near me, I still find myself in the subconscious reality that I had initially embraced those first days at the Kaiser Permanente Hospital, where the meanings and explanations of the illness continue to be parts of an animated film that I am not particularly interested in.

That's probably why, when Russell and Nik passed by to see how I was settling in, I talked a lot. I felt an urge to underline the positive aspects of my experience, and to tell them of my new ideas and perspectives. I snapped back into my old Martino character, the one that presented everything as just a possibility for creating stronger stories. Somehow I had to show them – as well as myself – how this experience had enlightened me, and especially, how I could use it to make our films, and our audience's lives, better.

I talked about *Bad Father*, Russell's *Happiness* documentary, and all the other films we had to do as soon as they had finished off fixing their movie *Arthur*. Russell and Nik, who were taken aback by my volubility, found themselves at a loss for words. Russell looked straight into my eyes and said, 'Mate . . . don't worry about all these things right now,' as Nik added, 'We've heard from different docs that you've been very lucky to even survive.'

After a pause, Russell said quietly, 'You could very easily have died.' And with his calmest smile, the one I had seen him use with drug addicts entering rehab, he told me, 'Take it easy. And enjoy your well-earned holiday, mate.'

The next day, Nicola, the bodyguard, Nik and Tom flew to New York with Russell to re-shoot some parts of *Arthur* (did I already tell you about their remake of the 1981 Oscar-winning comedy with Dudley Moore?). American audiences had loved Russell in his first couple of films and were ready to see him alone on screen. In fact, his team were so sure that *Arthur* would launch Russell into the stratosphere that they had flown me in to lay out and develop the next three steps of his career.

This was his ticket to the chocolate factory, and on the back of this, we would surely be able to set up a proper production company and start making big, radical Hollywood films ourselves. Once I moved here properly, I could start resolving some of my marital tensions, and perhaps even have enough calm to occupy my brain with its most recent sci-fi reality.

A few weeks earlier, I had accompanied Russell and his body-guard to the studios to see the first edited version of *Arthur*, with the director. I knew very little about the production, so I was mostly there as moral support and to give some external feedback. It's always difficult to see a rough cut of a film you have made. And now that Russell had married the queen of pop music, the personal stakes were even higher for him. He had invested so much time, energy and love in that project and now, in that little editing room, he would see the result for the first time.

Russell's reaction to the screening was very strong. While he went to the loo to think it through, I told the director that, from my outside perspective, I liked it. It was a version of Russell, as an actor, that I had never seen before. Up to now he had played mostly straight comedy characters, enlarged copies of himself, but here his character was both sweet and warm. When we got back to the car, Russell told us that he was generally happy with the film. We all agreed that it needed some changes, but as a first cut, it was OK.

A few days later, I realized that my perspective of *Arthur* and his economic reality was influenced by my own dreams and emotions. My opinion that focusing on 'sweetness and love' would heal any problems with this movie was definitely not how the producers saw it. They had invested more than $40 million and they were not going to accept that their film was not what they'd anticipated.

Although the executive producers had very different opinions about the film, they all agreed that *Arthur* was sick and needed an operation. The financiers, with scalpel in one hand and gun in the other, discussed all the possibilities and came up with a common strategy. When there is such an illness in your film, all the doctors will tell you not to mess around with new ideas, but simply to use what has been proved to work before.

I was not involved in this production, so I looked at these powerful people from afar, attempting to learn what was soon to be my job. I was new to this commercial world and I quickly realized that, first of all, you had to study the market. The comedy films that had made lots of money in the past few years were not warm and sweet; they surprised the audience with clever narrative structures that used every trick in the book.

The result of these financial discussions was that Russell and his crew moved back to New York, to resolve their creative battles with a re-shoot, while I and my whole family now had this wonderful house entirely to ourselves for three weeks. Down the street we had a gigantic and rather posh supermarket with fresh orange juice, sushi-style fish and good bread. One day, as Margarita was about to go out to buy some breakfast, she asked me, 'Do you want eggs?' and I snapped, 'You know that I can't eat eggs because of my cholesterol . . .'

This was the first time I realized that during my operation something had happened which was now influencing my mood and character. It was not at all like it was before; I was not the same. While I'd been insisting that I focus on 'normality', I had obscured the reality that everyone else was living. For a person who had just battled the attack of the Aliens and survived, I could take it easy and eat an egg with my family. I was sure that cholesterol wouldn't break out for one egg.

So I told my wife, 'Wait and let me put some shoes on. I'll come with you. We'll buy the eggs together.'

With our son Miro we walked down the street, opened the gigantic security fence and we left, on foot. It reminded me of our house in Rome, where we also had a fruit and vegetable market within walking distance. These houses in Los Feliz were extremely well kept and open and if I ever did encounter a person walking down the road, they were always fantastically friendly. As cynical as big city life is assumed to be, this wasn't it.

Miro ran ahead and blocked the sidewalk, yelling, 'Red light! Stop!' Margarita and I stopped and waited, watching each other, standing in front of a lovely blue house, until 'Green light!' was called. We passed by the next house and Miro called for another 'Red light!' which, once again, froze us in our step. I brought my hand up to touch Margarita's neck. For me she had always been the expression of a different world, an ancient culture where destiny and human bonds are ethereal. She understands love as a fusion of two souls and while I am with her, I am in touch with a secret, atemporal dimension that our culture has somehow lost.

This had never been part of my life or my education, but for her it was so obvious that in fact she could take it for granted. 'Green light!' We walked on and I looked up. It was February but the sun was shining and all the plants seemed to mock my concept of summer, autumn and spring. There doesn't seem to be any winter in LA and maybe there is no concept of death here, either. Who knows, maybe through the operation my universe has changed and I have landed in a parallel reality, where the spaceships have never actually landed on the moon, and where family fights and big dramas don't exist.

The next day, Margarita and I went to the Kaiser Permanente to meet Dr Vogel. He is one of those people who truly puts you at ease, which is great for a man whose profession is brain surgery. He asked me how I was doing and started taking away the metallic clips that were holding my head together. He was very proud of his work. It all looked good and I felt fine.

He clarified that he had only taken away eighty per cent of my illness, and that he had not gone any further, fearful that he might take away certain parts indispensable for speaking, thinking or reading. Since he was so friendly, we asked his advice on various possible healthcare and oncology options in the US, but as he told us of a few other good hospitals, he also said, looking at us sadly, that none of them would be cheaper or necessarily better than the one we were at. It all sounded fine to me. I was sure that somehow, we were going to make it.

In the days that followed, Margarita went back and forth to the Kaiser Permanente, picking up all the documentation on my illness. I soon learned that walking into a hospital with a wife who is a doctor herself gives the entry much more panache, and that other doctors would actually listen to her and even reply. Perhaps it is a certain tone that allows doctors to spot each other.

While on one side Margarita is a very pretty girl who takes hours to get ready and loves art and design magazines, on the other she is a super nerd who has obviously spent a ridiculous amount of time learning her trade. While I was still learning the ABC of my new world, she was trying to find me a way through the XYZ. I tried as hard as I could not to ask her endless silly questions whilst she was in her work mode.

There is a certain comfort in taking on the role of the happy idiot. Of choosing not to have the responsibility or knowledge to decide the next step of your life. While meeting all those well-dressed, tight-lipped professionals, I always tried to pull out my most cheery personality. They all knew that I did not understand what they were talking about, so from my very first entrance I would make sure to touch them with my hands and continue to look at their eyes, even if they were not looking at me. My instinct was that, as the character in centre stage, my role was to keep the optimism high, even when I was confronted with people whose job was to prepare me for imminent drama.

As a professional biophysics researcher, my sister Bianca knew how to put in funding applications. She was the only one of us who had both the technical knowledge and the patience to fill out these reams of text. I felt as if I had a crack team of top international experts working for me. I shared blood and soul with them and I wanted to make sure that I would not disappoint them. While their presence allowed me to stay calm and ignore the meaning of all those strange, dangerous, scientific words, I did sometimes feel that I needed to show them my physical and cerebral prowess.

One evening, during dinner, sensing that the energy of the crew felt low, I decided to tell them all the surreal tale of my day, as I was sure that it would cheer them up.

That morning, leaving Margarita at home to play with Miro,

my mother and I had been to a Citibank, where we had kept an account open since the 1980s. We were sure that if anybody could, they would be able to tell me my Social Security number. Focusing on Bianca and Margarita's eyes, I relayed the story: 'As Mom and I walked into the huge, open space of the bank, a young woman came towards us and greeted us with a classic corporate smile.'

For the delight of Miro, I did my best imitation of an insincere expression.

'She got us to sit down on these comfortable couches while we waited for one of the bank staff to go on their computer and find my name.'

Marianella raised her hand calmly and interrupted me, 'It must have been at least fifteen years since it was used. But we were sure that it was lying frozen in one of their computers, and as that smiling lady told us, once found, it would take only a few minutes for them to defrost it.'

I continued, 'The first name that the bank teller found was, obviously, Mom's, and then we had to sit down on our couches again and wait another ten minutes while she searched for mine. Impatiently, and very quietly, I told Mom,' putting my face right next to Miro, who was busy sticking his fork into his pasta and smiling, engaged by my physical performance, '"Mom, is it possible that a computer takes so much time to find a name?" And right at that moment, the lady called us back to the teller.

'When we arrived there, the face of our lovely bank teller looked shaken, and even a bit embarrassed. She was talking quietly to her colleague. They seemed confused. I was sure that I could help them if they let me. So I knocked on the window of the till,' as a sound effect, I banged my spoon on my glass. 'When her colleague had gone, she told me, "Mr Sclavi, from what I've found in our computers . . . You are deceased!"'

I looked round the table at Bianca, Margarita and Miro, who were all intrigued by now.

'I had given her my Italian passport and driving licence a few minutes before, so she must have realized that the big Italian dude in front of her was alive. Embarrassed, she turned to her boss, who, disappeared for a few minutes, then popped back out of his office and smiled at us.

'"Please accept my apologies. Is your father deceased?" I nodded. "Because most probably the two names and Social Security numbers have been confused in the paperwork, which would explain everything."'

At our living-room table, I raised my glass of water for a toast. 'I am legally alive!' I looked across at Bianca. 'We can finally use my Social Security number for our various submissions.'

Even though Margarita appeared to show interest in at least parts of my tale, she must have not really shared my dark humour. If truth be told, from the moment that I used the word 'deceased', I noticed that she was becoming more and more despondent.

While Bianca was putting Miro to bed, and my mother was washing the dishes, we went out for a walk in the mountains behind the house. I told her, 'I promise you that I am not going to die. It's a promise.' But as I looked for a reaction I realized that, for once, it wasn't about me. It was about her father.

She said, 'Today, while you were out, I Skyped with Dedo. He's talked to the doctors in Rome, who've told him and Jasmina to get their things together.' Tears started falling from her eyes. 'They told them that there's not much time left . . .'

While negotiating the scary realities of my drama, Margarita had not had a moment to think of the situation developing in that hospital in Rome. My arms were on her shoulders as the tears increased with every word. 'I miss my father . . .'*

---

* Margarita: 'His face looked skinny and tired. He continued to ask me about your prognosis and eventually I told him. It was that moment, as I saw his reaction on that computer screen, when I realized how bad it was. I heard later that my father, for the first and last time in his life, told his best friend, Uncle Rade, "I need to go to church . . ." He walked into that church and lit up a candle for you.'

Initially, Rome had seemed like a good place to find top-level cures for her father's pancreatic cancer, but now, without their daughter softly translating the oncological reality in Macedonian, the Italian doctors had given him and his wife Jasmina the raw truth of his diagnosis.

They were now on a flight back to their beautiful home in Skopje to embrace the inevitable, while their daughter was here, completely impotent. As she was trying to keep going, crying uncontrollably, I stopped her and held her in my arms as tightly as I could. I tried to share in her emotions, but I realized that I was just not able to be where she needed me. I was swimming up my own river, afraid that if I distracted myself for a second, I would choke.

~

Bianca and I walked through the hospital and checked into the finance office to give them my SS number and my 2010 Italian income tax return, which was very low. We were hoping to get some kind of discount at least. The year before I had worked mostly on developing projects with my London company, so apart from a few little advertising jobs, I had received very little income.

The woman put my details into her computer and said, 'OK, you fit into the group. And because you were checked in through the ER, you do not have to pay for the operation.'

You what? Really? Wow! Bianca and I walked out of the room in disbelief.

For that evening at least, we decided to ignore the fact that we had to put together enough dough to cover the costs of all the radiotherapy, chemo and the various drugs that I would have to take. We raised our glasses of juice to celebrate whatever had just happened, which I later realized was that I had fallen miraculously into that little gap of President Obama's brand-new Health Care Reform.

Keeping in mind that *Arthur* was to be released at the beginning of summer, I directed my attention towards finding a proper job, with an American company that was stable enough to allow me to pay for my cures. I needed to get back to work, to find a home for my family and a school for Miro. I knew that at some point Nik, the bodyguard and Tom would be coming back, and that we would not all be able to live with them. We looked for a new house in the same part of town, as most of our friends lived there.

I took myself to Adam Venit's office in the centre of Hollywood, and started talking at full speed about the various types of projects we should be looking at for Russell, and also perhaps a company that could give me a proper contract with some health insurance. When I stopped for a second to take a breath, I realized that he was sitting there with a half-smile on his face, looking bewildered.

Now that I think of it, the sight of me sitting there wearing my new German hat, talking enthusiastically about work, would have made anyone who had followed my tale from the beginning laugh (or maybe cry?). He hugged me, handed me a few screenplays that were potentially good for Russell, and we went out for lunch.

We met our wives at the restaurant across the street from his office. From the first time Margarita and Trina Venit met in India, they had determined that they were blood sisters, and seeing them sitting next to each other, so delighted with their friendship, brought me great joy. Even though I was surrounded by more Botox in that restaurant than I could take, it felt like everything was totally normal, to the point that it restored my belief that we were in the right place. Why could this not be our new normal, American life?

As the meal was finishing and we were waiting for the cappuccinos, Adam brought us to the main issue of the day, hospitals. Margarita stepped in with her professorial voice, telling them about all the information she was collecting about my illness and of her research for a second opinion. She added, 'There's also an old Macedonian friend of my father who is a professor at Columbia University, and maybe he can help us.'

As we had just avoided a bill for a hundred thousand dollars and had found a possible apartment near a good school for Miro, we were more than a bit optimistic that we would find a solution to all our problems right there in America. In hindsight, I wasn't the only person who did not appreciate the true extent of my illness. My mother was the one who had been leading our real-estate research and she had been wandering through the streets of our neighbourhood looking at 'For Rent' signs, while wearing a big, white woollen hat – a slightly odd fashion choice under the warm California sun.*

Margarita had started going regularly to an athletics club with Amanda Fairey, and I don't think I had ever seen her smile so often. Maybe it was just LA, but we were sure that everything was going to be fine. Did I say that already? It was all really too nice not to be fine.

Looking back at this period that we spent happily in Los Angeles, we must all have been drinking some strange 'health' cocktails, because we were plainly in denial of the gravity of the situation. When the first two of Bianca's applications for Health Insurance were refused, we started to realize that it was possible it was never going to work. Even if we all continued to put in our very best, we were not going to succeed. It was a simple matter of money. Of cash. Without a substantial amount of the stuff, we were lost. We had played all our cards and needed something else. Something creative. Something magical.

A few days later, Adam and Trina passed by to pay a visit, and brought us a couple of bottles of very good red wine. With my glass of juice in my hand, I noticed that they had

---

* Margarita: 'I remember that your mother would walk through potential apartments, saying, "Here is the terrace for Miro, here is the room for you, look at the view!" It was her way of defending herself from that moment and I was at peace with her. LA is such a beautiful place and we were all going to move there. Your doctors were good and we had to heal you there.'

both come with a very different, professional attitude – they were worried. One of Adam's partners had heard of my story and they told us that I should give him my full medical report and he would send it to the NIH in Washington DC, where his brother was one of the top managers.

The NIH, the National Institutes of Health, is the place where the smartest minds find solutions to the most complex problems. Although Margarita had grown up on the other side of the world, in socialist Yugoslavia, she knew that hospitals, like schools and everywhere else, always have a certain level of nepotism, and this could be a crucial breakthrough for us. Adam arranged for his assistant to come to our house and pick up all the necessary paperwork. They sent my assembled packages to the other side of America, in the hope of allowing me to take part in one of their clinical trials, and by doing so, be given the most advanced and pioneer cures without the millionaire prices.

Even if I was not completely sure that I wanted to leave this warm and calming land, I had to break out of my dream and my fictional spaceships, and concentrate on killing the real Aliens. While I was leaving behind my dear little cousin *Arthur*, whose illness was being cured in NYC with big money, my little family and friends might have just found me an exit from my own Catch 22.

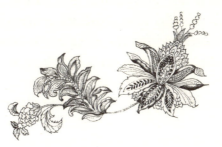

6

A Horse Race and Finding Love

Siena, Rome and Venice, 2002

I am sitting on a couch as I write you these words. Even if this particular one is a bit too floppy, after adding a few cushions, it does get into the right shape. I sat here for a good part of the last chapter and my back is still OK. I mention that because, over time, I have developed a unique relationship with couches: the sturdy ones, the floppy ones, and in particular those that fold out and become beds. There are important moments in my life when I have found solace from sleeping on different types of cribs.

Some people have tried to suggest that living on couches is shameful and, at times, late at night, I do understand where they're coming from. But I have also developed a deep admiration for the human experience that comes with staying with – or hosting – others. The energy of my friends, who have welcomed me into their houses, with whatever they have, has fundamentally helped me to get through all my battles with the Aliens.

This morning, as usual, I packed up my couch-bed, picked up Miro from his mother's house and walked him to school. Along the way, we stopped and had a quick chat with the crooked-eyed man who sleeps under the bridge. I believe that engaging with his sorrows, even if only briefly, is a part of life that is healthy for me, for my boy, and also for that man, to whom we brought a sincere smile (along with a promise of pizza later).

Now let's get back to my more historic tale.

~

It was 2002, and after having spent winter in Great Britain battling my comedian's drugbrella, I had taken a trip around Europe, staying on various friends' couches, licking my wounds and searching for any kind of work that could put my soul and economy back in order, until finally, in June, I landed back in Italy, in my family's house in Tuscany.

Villa Flora, with its gardens and animals, could have been the perfect place for me to relax and get back my strength after the defeat, were it not for the fact that it was the home of my Uncle Antonio. While it was big enough for every member of my family to have their own room there, ultimately the house was his – he was the one who had bought it, and he was the only one who lived there. And although it was not really my 'home', seeing how often I had changed houses, it was the place where I kept all my academic and fiction books, my records, CDs and almost all of my clothes. I have never thought about it that way, but yes, all my earthly belongings were there, in that lovely room in that beautiful house in the hills outside of Siena, and so it was the place where I felt most at home.

The fact was that I had not really lived in Italy since I was ten years old, when my father Gastone, who had studied chemistry and was secretary of the workers' union for the Italian chemical industry, received an offer from his counterpart in the United States to move there and so radically changed all of our lives.

Nearly twenty years later, the idea of returning to Villa Flora after the collapse of my company, which my uncle had surely heard about, generated more than a bit of stress for me. I knew that I was going to be confronted with the usual 'stop being a kid', 'get a proper job', and 'you are the idiot of the whole family'. The collapse of my first economically viable project was hard on me, and I did not need my uncle's constant commentary.

As I could not imagine myself trying to explain the story of Vanity Projects and its ridiculous dreams and its unavoidable collapse to him, I decided to cover up those professional burns by arriving at his house with a posse of female friends. I had told him not to worry, that they were all well-behaved grown-ups and I would be taking care of them, but as I got out of the car, his pair of exotic parrots started screeching from their cage, which scared some of the girls, who yelled even louder, and looking at my uncle I knew I had caught him in a really bad mood.

As we went in the entrance by the kitchen, he shouted at me in Italian then shoved a piece of bread and Parma ham into his mouth and walked past all of us towards his posh car outside. He hopped in and tried to tell me that he had too much to do with the Palio (the historical horse race), pointing his arm in the air as if to signal *Do whatever! Just get out of my way. I don't like, and I don't want to see, all those people in my house.*

This was a part of his character I was used to. While he behaved like this with most people, I felt that he had a soft spot for me, since I would occasionally manage to keep my cool and answer him calmly when he was criticizing me. I was not particularly worried at that moment, but I was left there having to explain the dynamics of my family to all my guests. So here is the story of the three brothers, which has always helped me to illustrate the complexity of loving the people who are closest to you.

Gastone Sclavi, my father, was born and grew up on the steep streets of Siena, and although his brother Antonio was somehow born only seven months after him, their characters could not be more different. When, seven years later, the third brother Fabrizio was born with one of his legs shorter than the other, his older brothers bonded and took care of him. Their family, of humble descent, stood up proud under the control of their mother, Zelinda. Yes, that is a funny name, with a funny story, because Zelinda's parents had already produced seven children, whose names all started with an A, so they decided to call it quits with their overgrown family and give their last child a name beginning with Z. Now Zelinda and her husband Aquilino worked hard in their new family bakery and made sure that their three boys could go to school.

In the early sixties, when my father Gastone moved to Milan to study engineering, there was great hope for him, but he gave up when he only had two exams to go before finishing his degree. There, away from the ancient little town of Siena, he had discovered other possibilities, something more important. A few of his friends in Milan had fought against the fascists and, like them, he wanted to contribute to a fairer economy and government. So when his friends persuaded him there were more useful ways for him to employ his engineering skills, he left academia and started a new life with the workers' union. This was a huge disgrace for his father Aquilino, who had been a member of the Italian fascists.

The times were changing and the city of Milan was the epicentre of modernity. My Uncle Fabrizio joined my father in Milan, and after doing an arts degree, he entered the world of fashion, where within a few years he was creating and selling

men's ties, and from there he became one of the youngest
editors of a glamorous men's fashion magazine.

My Uncle Antonio was the one who stayed in Siena and took
care of the Sclavi family's bread shop, which over time he grew
exponentially, almost to the level of a Sienese bread oligarchy.
Having risen from his father's humble condition to be a
successful businessman, and having become the president of
Siena's chamber of commerce, he needed to demonstrate his
newly gained status to the Tuscan aristocracy. It must have been
in the early nineties when Antonio found Villa Flora (the flower
palace). As soon as he saw it, he knew he had to buy it. It is
a proper seventeenth-century villa with a view of the city. While
for my Uncle Antonio this piece of real estate was his wife, his
lover and a symbol of his success, for the rest of us it was just
a great place to be.

Bianca and I, as excited teenagers, could not believe that our
family had become so wealthy. In the park there were outbuild-
ings for the two dogs and another for two horses. Horses? In
our family grounds? As soon as we told our American friends
about our new Italian base, it became a mandatory stop for all
their first-time trips to Europe. Our grandmother Zelinda had
worked all her life in the bakery and, even in her eighties, she
prepared food for all of us before going off to work.

She was the one from whose permission we asked when we
wanted to invite our friends. There were plenty of rooms and
so long as everyone behaved, she was always more than happy
to welcome them. As a good Catholic, one of Zelinda's rules
while staying there was that if you weren't married, you could
only share a room with someone of your own sex. What
happened in those rooms late at night did not concern her,
providing that in the morning, the house returned to its respect-
able state.

In the middle of the nineties, when my grandmother and
shortly thereafter my father passed away, the gigantic house
started to look as if it was overwhelming Antonio. He always

seemed to be frustrated by something, and as soon as we arrived he would welcome us by saying, 'Please don't stay more than a few days as it will annoy me. I'm not used to having people about.'

For someone like him, who had sacrificed a lot to be able to climb the social ladder of this ancient city, the idea that the family's line of succession was in the hands of the little Sclavi (me), who made his living mixing cocktails for a bar run by gangsters in Brixton, it was all deeply shameful. No matter what I had come up with, he was always very critical of my endeavours. My first films looked nice, but what about the money? He would often say, 'When I was twenty-two, I was already a university professor. How can you live without making money?'

A few months after the death of my father, Bianca and I were standing next to Antonio in the garden of Villa Flora, learning from him how to safely put a handful of seeds into a bowl to feed his two, rather angry, exotic parrots, when he told us that as both of us were obviously not interested in making proper money, or taking over the company, he was going to put together a fund. It was to ensure that, at the tragic moment when we would have the Villa and the bakeries in our hands, we would not have to sell it all immediately to cover the huge running costs.

As the birds were becoming excited, he quickly shut the door to their cage before continuing. He was impressed by the way that our father had raised us without making money the priority. For him, we both seemed well balanced and good-tempered and surprised him by never asking for cash. (In fact, he had got into the habit of handing it to us after every visit. We were both, after all, partly owners of the Sclavi bakery, so that money was actually owed to us, but if he needed to feel like he was giving us gifts . . . well, it was fine by us.)

While for people like my uncle, and I guess a good part of the western world, real estate is strongly associated with power and social success, I currently find it almost as stressful as oncology. Everyone I encounter ends up talking about it, and while some convince themselves that they absolutely need more, others – even in a time of crisis – sacrifice everything to hold on to what they have got. Once again, it is somehow felt disgraceful to show the world that you are moving backwards in your socio-economic standing. As the only economy that I should embrace in my current situation is one that keeps me calm, real estate feels counter-intuitive. But let's get back to my fun, historical psychodrama.

In the small town of Siena, where only 51,000 people live, everyone knows everything about everyone else, and the reputation of a family is extremely important. In my room on the second floor of Villa Flora, I kept a whole bunch of my father's classic clothes that I would only wear when I was there, to make sure I didn't make any unnecessary fashion statements in the town. Little details do quickly become a source of gossip in such places. Was I too baggy, too tight, too short or too colourful?

I have never managed to get my head around my Uncle Antonio's world or where his constant criticisms of the way I live my life come from. But I believe the unspoken reality behind all his frustration is that, while his brother Fabrizio was able to be openly gay in his fashion circle in Milan, Antonio has had to constantly pull a veil over his young homosexual partners. The centre of Siena is completely pedestrianized, so it is the perfect network for meeting people. Stopping along the way, Antonio usually introduced his young friends to the establishment as his 'cousins' or 'nephews'.

Clearly, since I was about the same age as his boyfriends, whenever he used to present me to members of other important Sienese families, he always emphasized the fact that I was his Sclavi nephew; and then, after shaking his head with half a smile, he would stress that I was almost thirty, and had not yet sorted out my life. I am sure that a good part of the town knew and recognized his young lovers, but in such a close-knit, conservative Catholic community the basic rule was to ignore those elephants walking down their street, and try to enter the main square, Piazza del Campo, as quietly as possible.

My original intention was not to surround myself with so many women in my gay uncle's house. They included Susan, Clair, Serife, Veronica, China, Jessica (and someone else whose name I don't remember), who had all become fast friends over a heavily alcoholic dinner at the lovely house I shared with Adrian Muys in London. Subconsciously, I must have made that whole crowd arrive there in Siena because I felt like an orphan of Vanity Projects, and wanted to hide away and lie in a warm, female embrace. But as I organized rooms for all my guests, I realized that I needed support. Without thinking about it too much, I picked up the phone and asked for assistance. My old friends Matteo and Giulio, who had both landed in the world of film production, were fans of the Palio and gladly agreed to come and help me with my 'problem'.

Siena is split into seventeen contradas, or neighbourhoods, and twice a year ten of them meet in the central square of the city for a bareback horse race, known as the Palio. This has been going on since the fifteenth century and people take it extremely seriously. The tradition is that if your contrada wins, you will celebrate for the rest of the year, but on the other hand, if your enemy contrada happens to win, you will live the rest of that year in disgrace. The winners pass through the whole city flying their flags and banging their drums, singing about their pride and mocking the shame you have brought to the town.

I grew up supporting la Lupa (the Wolf), who had not won a race since the Berlin Wall came down in 1989, and knowing that I really needed something to cheer myself up, I gave their horse full responsibility for my future. His victory would certainly boost my spirits, and give me faith. In the Palio there is a large quota of luck, but this time I was completely sure we were going to win.

The horses that take part in the race are selected by the city and then given to the various contradas through the spinning of a tombola. Furthermore, the position of the horses at the start – who is closest to you, and how close you are to the shorter route right of centre – is also decided by chance. Being given a horse who has already won a Palio greatly increases the probability of winning. This year we had landed the king horse, and we had hired the right man for the job. So I had good reason to feel optimistic and I would finally have a chance to see my Uncle Antonio truly happy.

As usual, on the day of the race, the city felt as if it was going properly mad. The members of each contrada walked with their horse through the whole city, accompanied by a crew dressed in wigs and clothes in the original fifteenth-century style. Aside from the poor animals, who are obviously excited by the drumming and singing, the focus of the parade is the two young men who show off their skills in shaking and spinning their flags dangerously close to each other up into the air. Tourists from every part of the globe push through the little streets to get a glimpse of this continuous show.

I met Giulio and Matteo in front of Il Duomo, the main church right at the top of the city, and introduced them to all my female guests. Both of them were thrilled to assist me in my endeavour. I had arranged with Antonio that I, and two of my friends, could join him in the window seat that he always rented for his guests. I chose Veronica, because she was simply too short and would get stepped on by the mob, and Serife, because I was sure she was going to faint under the scorching sun in the middle of the crowded square.

While Giulio and Matteo were getting to know my friends, my eyes were caught by a girl who seemed to fit there perfectly, sitting on the steps of the Duomo, the most beautiful church in the city, where black-and-white stripes adorn all the walls up to the highest view of Tuscany. While the crowd of tourists were snapping away at the various contradas with their colourful flags, my camera was only focused on her.

I grew up as a 35mm type of man so my first images of that

girl sounded like *cruncch* and then, as I loaded it back for a second look, *krrrick*. While the lower third of the photo showed a pair of short, tight blue jeans, the top third of the frame was dominated by her seemingly gigantic eyes, staring back at my lens. I was shooting in black and white, but I wasn't completely sure how to read her half-open mouth. Was it a symbol of surprise and curiosity – or perhaps her response to the photographer's frozen position?

I heard the unusual rhythm of the words coming out of her mouth while she was talking to her tall, blonde girlfriend, and when I realized they were part of a group of Giulio's friends, I approached and introduced myself in English. 'Is it the first time you've seen the Palio?'

In the chaos of the background noise, they smiled and nodded their heads. I said, 'Prepare yourself, as this sound will continue for the next three hours. It only stops when the horses come out,' but before I could ask them anything, I had to raise my hand in apology, as I was being pulled away by one of my lovely guests, who wanted me to explain to her about the contrada that was passing by.

Giulio and Matteo led most of my guests down to the square to find a good place where they were going to watch the race a few hours later. As I took my two visitors down a steep hill towards our window seats away from this chaos, I thought sadly that my camera would never focus on that girl again, but fortunately, halfway down, in the middle of the confusion, I spotted a face looking at me. It was her. She was sitting in front of a bar with her blonde friend, so I winged it. I told my two friends that this place had a good bathroom, and so they should use the opportunity.

While waiting I turned my head and smiled, as if I had just realized they were right next to me. I looked at them with my best 'surprised' face. 'I am impressed . . . I mean that you have found a place to sit in this mayhem. How do you know Giulio?'

The blonde girl seemed eager to talk, but as I tried to listen to her, I realized that my neck was subconsciously turning my head towards the left, where those gigantic brown eyes kept looking back at me, as if I had printed them on my heart the first moment that she appeared in my field of vision.

I told them, 'If you want to purchase one of the contrada's scarves, my advice is to get the ones of my contrada, the Lupa; they're black, white and red. They would look fantastic on both of you – well actually, I'm sure that anything would look good on you – but we do have the best horse and the best rider this year . . . and definitely do stay away from the Istrice, the Porcupine.' Unsure if they knew the animal that I was referring to, I raised my fingers next to my head and made an evil face. 'They are our enemies. They are bad . . .' Both of them smiled widely and nodded, as if they had heard this before.

As they were saying something to each other in a different language, I became aware of my American guests who had come back out of the bar, so I quickly said goodbye and walked away backwards with my hand raised towards the sky. With all my blathering explanations, I had not got any sense of where they were from, or even what language they were speaking with each other. Once we arrived at our window seat I realized that, once again, I hadn't even asked their names. I looked down on the crowded square, where everyone was slowly being squeezed together by more and more people, and called Giulio on his mobile, but it was impossible to get through with the continuous sounds of the bells and the drums, so I had to give up.

Considering how long the ceremony goes on for, the actual race is finished in one and a half minutes. If you are a bit distracted, you can easily miss it. That day, the worst thing that could happen . . . happened. It was not only the fact that the Lupa did not win, or that I was there with all these guests and I had raised their expectations, but that day l'Istrice, our arch rivals, won. They ran through the crowds screaming and singing their proud hymns, constantly reminding us that we, the Lupa, were the losers and that we had to take their insults for another year.

I tried to keep cool and joined my other guests, who were relishing this thrilling and emotional experience in the main square. In the middle of the horde, the girl suddenly reappeared for the third time. While I was distracted by our defeat and the general hubbub, she approached me and said with a smile, 'I am sorry you lost,' and then, following her group of friends, kept her eyes on me until her face slowly disappeared in the crowd towards the winner's celebrations. That was it. I had lost her forever.

~

A few months later – it must have been the end of August – while searching for a proper job in Rome, I decided to help a German director who wanted to shoot a short film there. I had to pick myself up from the destruction of my London life and somehow start to work. Whatever it was, I needed to produce something. That evening, I had set up a meeting with Giulio in Campo dei Fiori, to ask his advice on how to hire an Italian teenage movie star for my film, as she might possibly like to raise her reputation in English language countries.

I was aware that, at some point that evening, Russell was going to land in my life again. He had called me that afternoon, and I had heard his drugged-up voice half-laughing on the other end of the line, telling me cheerfully, 'I'm on my way to the airport. I'm coming to Rome . . . today!' My hope was that he was coming to get away from the bad influences in London and that perhaps, while he was here, I could do something to help him kick at least the worst part of his addiction.

While I was waiting for Giulio there in the square, it started to rain, and as I was looking for a place where I could shield myself, I saw the girl, the one from the Palio. Maybe it was her huge, dark eyes, or the energy of those horses running madly through the crowd, but I hadn't stopped thinking of her all summer. She was sitting alone in a famous Roman bar called I Pazzi – the Crazy – looking at the Romans running through the warm autumn rain. I stopped in my tracks.

For a second that seemed like an hour, I stood still and let the rain wash my hair. I passed by without stopping, acting as if I had an important place to be, and then our eyes met. Yes. It was her. She did see me, and she did recognize me. It would have been rude not to say hello, at the very least, so I walked back and approached her. I sat down and we started talking in English.

Where was she from? Had she told me in the chaos of the Palio? Just to be sure, I avoided that subject and let my big-ass smile lead me. She was drinking whisky and smoking a cigarette. A woman sitting alone in the middle of a rainy square in Rome drinking whisky is definitely not part of my usual narrative. She told me that she had just arrived from work at the Santo Spirito Hospital, and that she was studying there, but as I was getting drawn into her tale, the rain suddenly subsided and Russell re-entered my life with his usual panache, carrying a black umbrella as a walking stick. Upon seeing me sitting next to a beautiful woman, he moved towards us with his most wicked smile and predator eyes, using his umbrella like Gene Kelly in *Singing in the Rain*, or better still, like Charlie Chaplin.

I quickly made him understand, non-verbally, that she was not a welcome-to-Rome present for him. He realized that something was already cooking between us and so, a few minutes after introducing himself, he stood up and went in search of something else. Five minutes later, I turned around and saw him drinking merrily with a bunch of Brits, who were very excited to have encountered an MTV presenter on vacation. As Giulio arrived, he excused himself for his lateness and said, 'Great to see you, Margarita,' in Italian. I had forgotten that he knew her, and now, finally, I had her name.

In order not to lose her this time, I asked her to join us for dinner, at a nondescript Chinese restaurant nearby. In hindsight, I have to admit that the whole dinner was a big mistake, and it had nothing to do with a bad spring roll. While I had Russell on the left telling me about the evolution of Vanity Projects after my departure, and Giulio on the other side of the table giving me advice on my Roman production, I sat there only slightly hiding my disinterest. I couldn't care less. Margarita was probably a bit embarrassed by my attention, but she kept looking at me, so what could I do – apart from look back at her?

Russell's stay in Rome was relatively calm, in comparison to the constant chaos he had created in our London life. A couple of days later, I managed to meet up with Margarita in a bookshop and even though she was more than an hour late, I didn't seem to mind. While waiting there, I bought her a book by Trilussa, my favourite Roman poet, who wrote wonderfully in the Romanesc dialect, and signed it for her with a quotation from the poem 'Soap Bubble':

> The sky, the sea, the flowers and the trees
> seem to keep you company in flight.
> How do you manage so rapidly to seize
> all of the world's colours, all of its light?
> You take your pleasure in the world, and on
> you drift beneath the sparkle of the sun.

I hadn't even kissed her and I already knew that I was in love. The big, heart-bouncing kind. While most days I was producing and being first assistant director on that German film, in the evenings I tried to chase down Margarita, leaving Russell to have his own Roman adventures.

Russell and I were staying in the apartment of Vittorio Foa, my father's teacher and best friend. He had been put in prison in 1935 for his organization of an anti-fascist movement and so he remained one of the true Jedi Knights in my life. He was ninety-three and spent the warmer parts of the year at his house in the Alps, and so he gladly left his apartment to us.

One evening, after a long day of shooting, I came in and walked along the corridor to find Russell sitting on the corner of the bath wearing his Che Guevara underwear. He was smiling like a child after coming home from the park, where he had done something naughty. He was trying to clean his right leg, arm and hand. I guessed that something had happened while he spent the night out hunting for every possible drug in town. Giulio, with whom I had left him for safe keeping, had tried to bring Russell home on his scooter, but our distracted, exuberant drunk had not moved his body with the bike and, on a turn, had carried them both over on to the street; fortunately, with minimal repercussions for Giulio, his scooter, or Russell's legs. So, there in the bathroom, I told him the tale of this rush of love that was driving through my body.

In fact, I had never told him of my adventures while travelling through war-torn Yugoslavia in the early nineties and how, with my 35mm camera, I had tried to narrate the stories of those young people who reacted to that bloody war with stunning art and music. Margarita's character reminded me of the world I had discovered there, and the love for them which continued to ignite my soul. I had met Margarita three times already, and I had only managed to get one single kiss from her. I was going crazy.

Still in his Che Guevara underwear, Russell accompanied me to the kitchen to drink whatever we could find. Standing next to each other, with his hand on my shoulder to safeguard his scratched leg, we shared a dream, that in our lives we would find true love. The one that makes all other drugs irrelevant. The one that would give meaning to every day. The one that was now helping us to mend our messed-up friendship, which had been torn to bits by the collapse of our Vanity Projects.

~

A few days later, Russell left Rome and we both knew that he was headed towards the end of his journey. Either he was going to die doing something ridiculous, like throwing himself off a motorbike at speed, or his dear friend Heroine would gladly take that role, and convince him that there is no such thing as too much. Fortunately, later that year, Russell left his posh agent and met John Noel, who picked him up, like the father he never had, and dropped him into the Focus 12 charity rehab centre in Suffolk, the right place where he could find the only way out.

Originally, Rome was supposed to be merely a stop on my journey to find a film or a job that would give me some money, but surprisingly, in this strange town which I knew only from my childhood, I had found something different, something that I had neglected in my new career: I had found love. Of all the various people living in this extremely romantic location, I fell in love with a Macedonian. Now that I knew that my heart was beating, all I needed was a job. Something that could keep me close to her. I was in touch with some people in Italy who had liked the films that Emily and I had made, and I was sure that they could help to ease my entrance into their industry.

At the beginning of September was the Venice Film Festival, where I had a few crucial meetings with powerful producers, and I asked Margarita to join me on my trip to the Lido. I had hardly any money, so I booked us a room in a monastery next to one of the most beautiful churches in Venice. As it was a proper monastery, I had to tell the nuns that we were married and that we would obey their rules and come back to our room by 11 p.m. We were just starting to get to know each other and Margarita must have found my choice of lodging more than a bit odd. I guess if you have been raised under Tito's regime, the idea of living with nuns on your first night in a 'hotel' would be . . . unfamiliar. Fortunately the view out of our window was simply priceless and the weather was stunning, which allowed Margarita to throw herself into my adventure.

In the Lido, where the festival takes place, I chased up my contacts until finally I met Marco Muller, who was chatting with one of his film directors. As I was asking him for advice about the producers I should meet, he stopped me in my tracks and told me that even though he didn't have much money, he had just won an Oscar for the Slovenian film *No Man's Land*, and had closed a three-movie deal with Rai Cinema, and so would gladly offer me a job in his newly founded company in Bologna.

That night, I met Margarita for dinner, and with the biggest smile on my face told her, 'I'm not much for games of chance, but you've brought me quite a bit of luck, and I'm not going to let you disappear again from my life.' On our way back to Rome, we stopped by Bologna, where I was going to work from then on. Margarita met Muller and all my future colleagues, and she told me that she found it all very exciting. Everything was coming together perfectly. Or so I thought.

When I went back to London to pack up the remnants from Vanity Projects and bring them down to Bologna, Margarita withdrew from all contact. I was bewildered, my emotions in disarray. For quite a few years, text messages had been a normal way of communication for me, and I had sent her several stories hoping to get a reaction, or perhaps just to cheer her up if she was having a bad time with something out there. What could have happened? On 26 September, I sent a big bunch of roses to the psychiatric ward of the Policlinico hospital, hoping that I could at least reach her for her birthday. The phone rang and I finally heard her voice, but patients or other doctors must have been nearby, because her tone was very formal, as if I was a nuisance who was pestering her.

When I returned to Rome, I eventually managed to arrange a meeting with her. I was half-worried and half-angry, as she was making my fragile little heart bounce up and down a bit too much. As she arrived at the bar, with what had become her classic forty-minute delay, I looked into her huge eyes and wanted to fall asleep in them and dream forever. With just a smile, she managed to make all other problems seem inconsequential. It was confusing. She responded to my various queries with stories about other women wanting to kick her out of the country, for some reason that I didn't comprehend. There was something I was forcing her to say, that she was actively trying to avoid answering.

As a provocation, I threw into the air the question, 'Is there another man?' She sustained that pause for what seemed like forever and I had to accept that she was not going to reply, unless I continued guessing. When I finally spotted her lie, I realized that it had been there from the very beginning and, driven by excitement, I had decided not to see it. As soon as it was in my head, it made me think back over every moment we had spent together.

In a moment of enlightenment, I understood that was probably the reason why I'd had such a hard time getting a first kiss from her. I paid the bill and left her with the remains of the last bottle of wine, and, drunk and full of sadness, I went alone to a hard-core, techno-music club to dance my sorrows away.

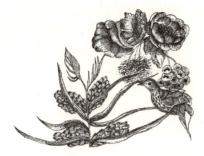

7

From LA to DC

Washington DC, 2011

I was sitting there in the garden of our beautiful house in Los Angeles with my eyes shut, contemplating the beauty of winter, when my phone rang. It was the voice of the top professor at the National Institutes of Health, the foremost US Government health research facility, known as NIH. They invited me to Washington DC to undergo a series of tests to establish if I, or my illness, was cool enough to take part in their experimental radiotherapy. I was slightly shocked that such an elite research institution would be interested in me: I was always a decent student, but never the top one.

I remember that when Cambridge University accepted me for graduate economics, I was stunned. I thought that a place like that would accept only the top students and they had chosen ten of them . . . and me? I, who had never got an A or A+ or A++, was accepted with the top students? In fact, written at the end of my Cambridge University acceptance letter there was a small detail. I had to send them documents from Berlin University proving the research and work I had claimed I had done there. If I was able to deliver it, I would be allowed into that Ivy of all Ivies institution and be drinking whisky with the future leaders of the world.

There are thousands of children who grow up wanting to be pilots of a spaceship, but only very few make it. Although Bianca was now back in Paris nurturing her bacteria, I was backed by my crack team of Dr Margarita, conflict-resolution master Marianella, and the cutest boy in the world as our mascot, we were going to get me into that NIH 'Spaceship'. I didn't completely understand what would happen there, if I did get in, but the hope was that this new kind of radiation would give me a few months longer, and everybody around me seemed very focused. Up until now the NIH had accepted only twenty-two people to enter their version of the NASA elite, so if I managed to get in, I would be only the twenty-third person to undertake such a journey in their Spaceship.

Our arrival in Bethesda, close to Washington DC but in a different state, it turns out, was a climatic and emotional shock, aside from what I was about to go through. From sunny and beautiful LA, we landed in the cold, harsh winter of the east coast. When I went to meet Dr Howard Fine in his little room on top of the huge NIH building, he was perfectly charming. He told me that he would like me, or my brain at least, to be part of one of their Spaceship test cases, which all sounded stupendous, until he confirmed that it was all dependent on my passing some tests.

What can you do when the tests are health-related? Do you try to look particularly sick? Or particularly healthy? Can you do anything to influence the result, or is it one of those rare occasions where your body will give completely 'objective' replies to their questions? I calmly assumed the latter. In the same way that I had not consciously invited the Aliens to enter and attack my brain, I would not be able to influence any test score. Or so I thought. And that was my first experience of how medicine is a much more creative art than we think.

After two days of tests I was told that one of my results was too high and that I could not be accepted. No free health care. No top-rate doctors. All because I failed some of their tests? I was told that they would redo the blood test the next day, but it was improbable that I would get it.

At seven o'clock in the morning, I received a phone call from the assistant of the big, world-class professor, who told me, 'If you want to get into the trial – and the big doctor would like to have you – come here in one hour, without having urinated and having drunk two full Diet Cokes.'

There were no discussions, comments or doubts, and in that silence everybody moved to war-zone rhythm. The Diet Coke was bought, we all got dressed, and while I was drinking my fizzy solutions to free medical care we headed to the NIH headquarters.

I could not believe that I was putting so much trust in the effects of that carbonated drink, and its magic serum that could open the door to that hyper-scientific world. It was simply ridiculous. Even if the magic potion within those products could make a difference, it would never have enough power or time to get from my mouth to my blood.

By that point I didn't care. I just wanted to get them the blood they wanted, to go to the bathroom and pee. I did my job and then we waited nervously. Did I do enough? I felt responsible, but didn't quite know what I was responsible for, or what I could do to make this a success. Even though there was continuous quarrelling between my mother and Margarita, I had the sensation that we were all a team, we shared an aim, and that I could not disappoint them. A few hours later, I got the phone call from the assistant. My result was eighty-three, instead of the one they needed, eighty or less.

What a blow! We had put all our energy and hopes into the success of that blood test and failed. It was perhaps the most abstract challenge that any of us could have confronted, but nevertheless . . . somehow we all felt we had failed. What could I have done better? What would have happened if I had drunk full-energy Coca-Cola or even Fanta for that matter? If it was sugar that I needed, maybe Sprite would have done the trick.*

Was it possible that in the middle of the night I'd had a dream of being in a boat splashing through the sea, and sleep-walked my way to the bathroom, and so ruined it all? Could I really have done that? Considering that this was the most important test in my life, how come I had failed?

Initially, I didn't even know if I believed that taking part in this trial was what I wanted to do. I didn't like this city. LA had been kind to us – why couldn't I be in California? There, between the warmth of their winter and the daily battle in my head, I had somehow found peace. We felt welcomed by our friends, and sitting in their garden, there were moments watching the kids play when time seemed to stand still, and I admired my fortune.

A few more moments like this would surely be worth more than a lifetime of fear, anger and stress. Stopping this war would not necessarily mean giving up, would it? I could face acceptance with clarity and peace. I had never thought of

---

* Blood sugar levels increase dramatically within twenty minutes of drinking the fizzy drink, the artificial sweeteners causing a spike in insulin.

looking for a good place to die, but actually, a place with a view of the Pacific Ocean could be all right.

As these various defeated thoughts ran through my head, my beloved family was already packing its bags in our tiny hotel room and our three-year-old was playing with his train between the beds. He raised his head as he arrived in the station, and as our eyes met he smiled at me for a minute, until the 'dang dang' of the station pulled him back on route. I heard a phone ring from my bed and the top professor himself was on the line. He told me, 'I can't do anything with these results. I do need eighty on your blood test to accept you. Drink all the liquid you can and come again tomorrow morning.'

We had all been sitting in this small, cramped hotel room and running around doctors' offices for days, and none of us wanted to give up: we wanted to fight for victory.

'I'll go and get some water . . .'

What can I do? Drink, I guess.

That morning I took the bus to the research centre, which had become my normal routine in these three short days. It was inconceivable that we would no longer go there. We crossed the entrance way, traversed the military-style security and finally got to the familiar building, number ten. The top building. The architectural vanity of such a space proved its power. Upon entering the thirteen-storey building, one was embraced by the postmodern architecture and all its windows and lights. The spaces were wide and the elevators plentiful.

The walls of the entire entrance hall were covered with large photographs of the various presidents of the United States touring the facility, and asking questions with great interest. This is the power. This is my safety. This is the truth. Please take my blood again, make it be good and then let me go pee!

My work was done and we sat around in our tiny room arguing with each other. Knowing that, most probably, our experience here in Bethesda was finished, we disagreed about the next step to take. Should we contact that person or the other one? That doctor, or the one who is a friend of our friend? Who is better? Would it mean that we'd have to move to Milan? Or to Bologna? Our son was ignoring his cartoons, and making the trains roar with power. The phone rang and the assistant spoke. She opened her mouth and told me, almost incredulously, that this time my results were exactly eighty. Eight zero.

Usually, these kinds of results don't change like that. Just a single number more would have meant failure. But it was zero, and we were in. Free health care. Free from our fights about where would be the best place to go. Free from the divisions and, for a moment, in that tiny room we had harmony. We were in America and WE'D WON!

For that split second, the Aliens were defeated, and my brain was stretching its bones in the expectation of imminent resolution. Like getting into Cambridge or having a healthy child or winning the lottery. From now on, no one could take this away from me. The details of this treatment were not clear to me, but by looking at the smiles of my family, I felt that I had increased my probability of life.

I went in to meet my whole new team. My radiologist was obviously 'the best' at finding innovative ways of radiating my head. He was the peacock of his department, and from his tone of voice I realized that he was so experienced and powerful that I was not going to see him very often. He introduced me to his crew, who I would meet with every morning, five days a week, and who would lay me down in their Spaceship and bomb the hell out of my brain.*

Since our next meeting was in another building, Margarita and I wandered about the city of the NIH, which seemed like various small towns. After getting lost a few times, we arrived

---

* Margarita: 'While waiting for an appointment with Professor Fine in Bethesda, I started talking to a woman who was obviously living a very similar reality and she told me immediately that I was going to need a back-up. A community. A therapy group to support me. I understood it, but I did not really embrace the importance of that advice.'

at our destination and laughed, because it looked more like an art studio than a scientific research centre. The nurses laid me down and asked if I liked my haircut. I had not cut my hair or beard since I woke up bald in LA, and yes, I had thrown away the hair that Russell had kept for me.

It was cold in DC and I had received two cool hats from friends in Europe, so I didn't understand the nurse's comment, particularly in this environment. In fact, I was feeling quite cool with what hair I had on my head, and I was delighted that it had almost completely covered the scary scar on the left side.

The thing was this: they were going to make a plastic mould of my head, with my face pointing up. I would be wearing that white mask every time I lay down in my Spaceship. Its purpose was to keep my head in exactly the same spot every time I was there, so that all the machines could continue accurately hitting the Aliens who had squatted in the left side of my brain.

I realized their question about my fashionable haircut was justified. From that point on, I would no longer be able to cut my hair. One of the two nurses looked at me and said, 'You are aware that you're most probably going to lose some of your hair in this process, and that you're not going to be able to cut it to make it straight?' I paused for a second and thought, so what?

After a few more stops I was introduced to my nurse, the person who was going to accompany me throughout the whole adventure. She was a fifty-year-old woman who at our first encounter greeted me with a big smile and a *'Benvenuto!'* She was from a classic Italian-American family and exuded warmth and emotion. I was so relieved that, in the midst of those sophisticated professors, I had actually found a magical person who would be taking care of me from then on. Every week she would be measuring my weight, checking my blood results, and generally taking care of any anxieties that I had with reassuring tales of previous patients now starting to run marathons.

Even if they are never directly remunerated for that part of their work, nurses are the secret psychologists of any hospital.

They know how to listen, they let you cry with no comment and leave you be when you need to be alone. In the larger band of the hospital, the nurses are the bass players. While the doctors are there showing off their guitar riffs and the surgeons shake their booty like peacocks, the nurses keep everyone grooving and hold the rhythm of our hearts. I am very sad that my brain no longer holds the names of almost anyone of those wonderful people, but if I ever did find a way to see them again, I would love to give them all a bunch of flowers and a big hug.

As Margarita and I were walking out of the research centre, I received a phone call from Adrian Muys, my corporate consultant friend, whom I had lived with in London when Vanity Projects collapsed. He had found us an apartment in what he said was the best neighbourhood in town. Anything would be better than that tiny room in the hotel, which just squeezed our fragile souls together. We packed our bags and headed towards the gay district of Washington DC. It was on the metro line, which five days a week would bring me to the NIH in suburban Bethesda. Finally, things were going our way.

We wandered through that three-storey house, covered with tasteful art and filled with beautiful furniture, feeling happy, really happy. Margarita's American phone kept on ringing, but as often happened, it did not connect. The kitchen was fully furnished and even had a lemon squeezer (you know, one of those ones designed by . . . *thanks, Alex, for that* – Philippe Starck). The beds were already made and, looking at each other with a smile, we chose our favourite room on the third floor, where we could sleep with some privacy.

The first place we had lived together was a rented apartment near the Vatican, where we had dreamt of a house of our own in which we could paint the walls as we wanted. We instinctively shared an excitement for interior design, so here, far away from nuns and priests, and far enough from my Spaceship in Bethesda, we had landed in our fantasy house. The owner, an older, gay man with Italian ancestry, was ready to give us the keys on the spot. With no hesitation, we took it.

We walked outside to look at the house and check on Margarita's phone. Suddenly it rang again, the shrill sound making her jump. The conversation that followed in Macedonian was replaced immediately by high, hysterical sobbing. Margarita's father, Dr Stojan Aleksievski, had died at the age of seventy-two. As I held her in my arms as tight as I could, I realized that I had been completely neglecting her. Whilst I had been focusing all my energy on getting into the American oncology VIP room, I had lost touch with her father's fight with his own Aliens.

Our bags were still in Adrian's car, so we all piled back in and started our long ride towards the airport. Aside from holding her tight, there wasn't much I could do to assist my wife.

Stojan was the professor and head of psychiatry in the state hospital of Macedonia, and we were a funny couple when we walked about together. He was physically quite a bit smaller than me and even though English was not his favourite language, he always made an effort to find the words that would allow us to understand each other. In the moments when we could not really communicate, he somehow managed to find comedy. His tragic and earnest tales of his extremely ill patients usually ended with him raising his hands as a sign of accepting the limits and the drama of our lives, but just as quickly he would sit down at his piano and by singing us a variety of Slav and American jazz classics, cleanse our souls and elevate our mood.

Aware that I had some difficulty following the alcoholic rhythm of Slavic men, on social occasions, rather than embarrassing me, he would move his hands over my glass and pretend to refill it. Throughout her education, Margarita had followed her father's trail, and even if he was obviously disappointed to have lost his top student to Italian psychiatry, Stojan remained curious and continuously engaged with his daughter in discussions of new strategies to assist these excited and troubled brains.

After that seemingly endless car ride to the airport, I put

my wife and son on the first flight to Skopje, which, for them, must have been a journey to the other side of the world. Now our beautiful three-storey house seemed bare. The empty rooms, the well-designed walls, all felt too funereal. In my joy of getting into those research trials, I had also forgotten the sad reality of all of those people in America who had gone back home and, with their families, had to accept the inhuman cost of private health care.

I'm fortunate to have grown up reading comic books and in these moments they truly did save the day. In the middle of 1990 I got addicted to the *Sandman* comics series by Neil Gaiman. They might be perceived by some to be strange stories for nerds and stoners, but when it comes to a world lacking in religion, they rock.

Gaiman's representation of Death is very different from anyone else's idea of the grim reaper. She has very pale skin and deep black hair. She looks like a beautiful teenager, who decides to be radical and wear only black. I am sure you have all encountered them somewhere. I think they are called Goths, but I must remember to ask Alex to help me double-check that word.

As I would no longer have the reassuring body of my wife next to me when I woke up in the middle of the night, and there would be no sound of my boy dreaming with his hands up over his head, my memories of such fictional characters would be useful. Knowing that the aim of Death in many stories is surprising and unexpected, allowed me to let her escort me up the stairs and choose one of the empty rooms where I would now be lying alone. Generally, Death smiles at everyone and brings calm to those whom she accompanies into her world. Crucially for me, in a few of her adventures, she engages with characters who do not end up dead.

~

A few days before, Margarita and I had talked with the big doctor (*come on, Alex, you should really try harder and remember his name*) about our plan to have some more children. He had looked at us firmly and told us that this radiotherapy was going to have a radically negative effect on my sperm and, as far as he was concerned, the only safe way for us to conceive was to put my sperm in a freezer before I started the therapy.

There are still places, both in America and in Europe, where due to religious convictions you cannot find a parking spot for your sperm. Fortunately, Adrian Muys, my gigantic little angel in this adventure, offered to accompany me to one of the four states that surround DC where sperm banks are allowed.

So Adrian picked me up from my new house in the gay part of town, and off we went. He had his camera in the car, as this was going to be the beginning of a story that would document me while I was going through the experimental trials.

We were going to begin by filming me leaving sperm in a plastic box, and all the emotional, tragicomic implications this entailed. Sadly, as soon as we arrived at the lab an hour away from DC, and we sat down in that big corporate office to fill out the necessary paperwork, a member of staff stood up from his table and put his hand in front of Adrian's camera. Filming was not allowed anywhere on the premises.

This extremely simple process was quite expensive considering that they only asked me for one dose, one . . . splurt, which they were going to keep in storage for me. The rental space for that dose was something like $700 a year, which is more or less the same as I would have to pay for a private parking place for a car. I was going to do this for Margarita. I put her name on all the documents, so that she could access my sperm whenever she wanted and without my presence.

Which, for me, is by far the strangest entity that anyone could ever inherit. A new child, a little brother or sister for Miro, could be conceived with that little plastic box, even after my death. It made sense, and I appreciated the prudent choice by Margarita (who does not usually think this pragmatically), and in any case, I understood the rationale, even as it kept feeling odd to me.

My mother, who had obviously been extremely anxious,

finally found a measure of reassurance in our new researchers and now that Bianca was about to arrive, decided she could go back to Milan and rescue the various projects that she had been ignoring in the past few weeks.

I was becoming aware of my own reality, and particularly of my impending end. I started to notice that my psychological fight for optimism was expressing itself throughout my body. I felt tired and did not want to share the thoughts that were in my head. But once my sister Bianca, the calmest and most focused person I know, arrived from Paris, the energy levels and mood of the house fundamentally changed.

When we were kids, our father Gastone had always kept the house filled with classical music, from Mahler to Shostakovich, but as a good older sister, Bianca had been introducing me to the better parts of eighties music. We had grown up in Italy until the early eighties, when my father moved us and our mother to the United States, where he had been offered a job in the chemical industry.

Ten years later, when my parents came back to Italy, Gastone said in an interview, 'What I was doing in America was frontier exploration. I worked on biotechnology, particularly on polymers and ceramics. I bought three companies and closed two others. It has been a fascinating and complex experience.'

In fact, I remember as a teenager watching Bianca and him working together on sophisticated recipes in the kitchen of our house in Westchester, New York, and for me that already looked like scientific research. She obviously followed my father's calling.

Ever since she left home and went to Reed College, on the other side of America, we have remained quite distant from each other. While she was in her world of pure science, I had embraced the differently complex reality of political science. Even after the arrival of email, we were not much for chit-chat. We sustained our sibling bond by sending each other mix tapes, then mix CDs, to introduce each other to new worlds.

Now, after so many years apart, living together in Washington DC felt extremely normal and comfortable. As Bianca knew from her scientific world of bacteria, staying calm and eating well is a crucial part of any experiment. She had brought with her a whole stash of new and old music for me to rediscover, and with that I found a certain peacefulness. The natural rhythm that guided our every day even allowed me to explore some of my more frivolous and childish scientific philosophies. Not easy, considering how much stress had been growing in my broken brain. You will encounter my mental explorations shortly, as they became crucial parts of my radiotherapy.

Every morning, after travelling on the underground to Bethesda, we walked through the high-security gates and within five minutes we would arrive at building number ten and walk to the elevator past the presidents' photographs hung along the walls.

From the first time we arrived, and the lift door opened in the −1 level, I felt a strange energy, something like jumping into a boat, parked in a land-locked city. This was no place for claustrophobics.

There, in the underground waiting room, the first person we met every morning was an obese secretary, who, after introducing herself the first time, never spoke to me again. She was quite a bit bigger than whatever chair she was sitting on, and every morning after picking up the phone and saying, 'MARTINO SCLAVI has arrived!' continued typing away at her computer, simultaneously keeping an eye on the discussions of the ladies on a daytime TV show on the screen that hung high up on the wall.

Bianca and I were usually still half asleep when we sat down in the seats under the television set, and while my sister typically opened her backpack and pulled out copies of articles that she had brought with her, to continue following the developments of her crew in Paris from afar, I tried to stay calm and keep the bad thoughts of the rampaging Aliens away from my head.

When I am forced into places and situations like that, where I can smell and observe similarly ill people, openly distraught and lost, who are wandering around me, I usually find myself thinking of being in an 'Aliens' type film. My use of the word 'Alien' while talking about my cancer is a conscious creation of fiction, and I have heard that it occurs in many similar patients. Or at least the younger ones who have mostly experienced death through films.

And if that does not work for me, which is usually due to the stress that is attempting to overwhelm my body, then somehow I have to release the pressure. Even in public. I have to close my eyes for thirty seconds, open them, close them again, start thinking of my mantra, and then meditate to clean my brain of all thoughts. In particular, the ones about my imminent death.

And all such details. The only time that meditation does not work is either when there are people yelling around me, or I start feeling the arrival of a headache. Then I have to ask whoever is around to help me find a place where I can sleep a little bit. Yes, I have become an expert napper, I can do it anytime and anywhere. Recently I have even found myself falling asleep on a very small baby's bed.

From the very beginning, the two men who ran my machine seemed to be following a strict protocol, and did not look as if they were up for any chit-chat. They just laid me down, fixed my head firmly in its position, covered it with its plastic copy, walked out of the room and turned off the light. I closed my eyes, and upon hearing the first blow of the loud sound, I crossed the threshold of reality. Fortunately, I also had my sister's eighties music stuck in my head.

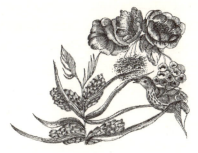

8

My Trips in the Spaceship

Washington DC, 2011

Having my sister nearby made it possible for me to enter that Spaceship to the rhythm of Lenny Bruce's comedy and the music of R.E.M.'s 'It's the End of the World as We Know It (And I Feel Fine)'. I was not only 'feeling fine', I now also had a guide to illustrate the adventures as they were developing in my brain.

This is what happened in my mind during those trips in the Spaceship.

The first things that I would encounter were bacteria. During our sleepy chats early in the morning, sitting on the train from DC to the NIH, Bianca had been telling me their stories and the fact that it was indeed bacteria who were the first creatures in our world a few billion years ago.

I realized that I had been walking around whistling to the stars without knowing that I could see only a fraction of the reality that is around me. We never think that there is a micro-universe inside us, or inside all the plants and animals. Those invisible creatures are an essential part of life, and if we mess with them, there will be repercussions. Without any need for Twitter or *Huffington Post*, they are in constant communication with our body, and they are all working and collaborating together.

The success of one is the success of everyone. In fact, the activity of the bacteria inside us can affect the strength of our immune system, and even influence its ability to fight against Aliens. Sadly, many of the medications that are made to combat Aliens also end up affecting the inner bacterial ecosystem and thus create a whole series of other problems. Often, in these oncological realities, even if the bacteria are focused and trying to be a team, the final result is that they fragment and watch each other disappear.

What can I do about this? The risk of not taking my medication is too high, according to the current state of scientific knowledge, so I have to try and help my bacteria to stay fit somehow.

To defend the complex world of the microscopic bacteria, I need to care, to give a shit about how they respond to music or food or my mood. If we were clever, we would prioritize the millions of microscopic creatures and let them lead our universe. If the bacteria are at war with various Aliens, we must make sure we are feeding them the right stuff, and not stressing them with the work it takes to digest a cheeseburger.

Think of the sad little bacteria all confused about dealing

with the Aliens on one side and the burger on the other. I have never met an oncologist who cares about my diet. I understand their chief priority – and it is a pretty big one – is to help me kill my Aliens, or at least keep them at bay; unfortunately they never seem to consider what is happening to the bacteria in my belly, while digesting heavy food or taking anticancer drugs. I guess that my sister is the only person I know who can read scientific reports about diets and knows how to judge their veracity in each particular case.

The only way I have to understand this social dynamic within our body is to compare it with our new vision of the environment. Recently, we (the population of the so-called more developed countries) have entered a new paradigm of collaboration and understanding with nature, where we have become conscious that each mistake we make has a repercussion in a different part of our world.

Every piece of garbage that we throw away will have an effect on our environment at some point, and similarly every piece of garbage that we put in our body will have an effect on our inner ecosystem. At times, it is the same piece of garbage – such as pesticides – that does both.

Since this relationship between our microscopic bacteria and the environment around us was too complex for my little cut-up brain in its Spaceship, I found refuge in a world that I knew something about, cinema. For me the success of the film *Avatar* teaches us that we must learn to have a relationship with the environment, that we are part of an ecosystem. Those fictional creatures from that foreign world showed us that in order not to focus on money and greed, we need a belief system that brings our priorities together.

If I, like millions of people, have been able to follow the doctrine of God, or Jesus Christ, who we cannot and have never seen or touched, then I am sure we can all try to have a relationship with the practically invisible creatures that live within our bodies.

If the pharmaceutical industry, for example, put some time and investment into advertising the importance of bacteria. Or if every Wednesday at lunch we all joined together in a big place like a hospital, where people are trying to fight the righteous war in their bodies, and prayed to the bacteria, while asking them what we can do for them. What kind of exercise should we do, what food should we eat? We could be opening up the doors to let the body live for as long as it has strength, and die when it is tired of living, not when it is unable to respond to the attacks of Aliens or their friends in McDonald's.

Or, as Russell says, 'Our eyes can only see between infrared light and ultraviolet light. There's light bouncing around everywhere. Our ears can only hear a tiny decibel range; we can't hear the noise of a dog whistle, can't hear any high-pitch frequency sounds. Isn't it likely then that there are other vibrations, frequencies, energies and types of consciousness moving through the universe?'

~

I would walk out of those trips in my Spaceship, raise my hand to say goodbye to the obese lady at her computer, and take the lift back into reality with Bianca. I usually bought a cup of tea and tried to get my zonked brain back in order, before attempting to talk to anyone. That last radiotherapy trip must have opened up a gap in my head, because I found myself asking my lovely nurse what other activities I could explore while I was there, in the gigantic building number ten, and with no hesitation she organized a set of meetings for me with different doctors and specialists.

My first appointment was with a hypnotherapist. I'm fairly sure that were it not for the discussions with my sister running through my head during those radiotherapy trips, I would never have agreed to embrace such ideas. As soon as I met that professor, I almost laughed. He wasn't acting a part, he really was Ned Flanders, the neighbour in *The Simpsons*. His voice and his smile seemed way too cheery for the design of that building, and because of that he immediately put me in a good mood.

He was a big deal professor, as I guess were all the people working at the NIH. Upon my first meeting with him, I told him, just to be open, that at least up until now I did not believe in what he did. I had always thought of hypnosis as a magic show, where the whole thing depended on a fundamental trick. He did not seem to mind my doubts, as he must have been used to this attitude. He just continued to speak to me with his slow and very clear voice, and unlike all the other professors there, he spoke directly and firmly.

From our very first meeting, I liked him and felt as if I wanted to hang out with him. I sat down on his electronic couch, where I repositioned myself almost to a sleeping position. He turned off the main lights and started talking to me calmly. There were no tricks, but somehow I got carried away with his calm voice. I started visualizing my brain in its physical essence, and imagined my cancer, as if I was controlling it and moving it out of my head. It was an extremely 'cool' experience, different from anything I had ever done, and it did not require me to do anything particularly stressful, so I asked him to please book me as many meetings as possible.

~

After travelling through this parallel world of radiotherapy for a few weeks, I started to understand my life and the bacteria as part of an interconnected reality. It is like a flock of birds flying in the sky, following a groove together that they are all creating.

To understand a complex system, you have to appreciate that all the components relate to each other. Once you start with this, you can assist the straightforward world of mathematics and allow it to be coherent with other arts like yoga or hypnotherapy. The clearest and most explicit way I have seen this work is the difference I felt when I started to drink fresh green juice in the morning and cut out sugars. Such a small change produced a large effect on the type of energy that I lived with, resulting in a new balance in my body and moods. As the doors open, the options are endless.

In order to speak this new language, I have to focus on the rules of interaction. Networks are ideal representations of our complex system, where the links are given by their communications. In order to accept this, first of all I have to come to terms with the fact that cancer actually forces changes in the expression levels of hundreds, if not thousands, of different genes within our cells.

As my Professor Fine is attempting to prove with all these experimental trips that I am doing, cancer susceptibility and progression depends upon the emergent properties of many genes, each of which individually has a small effect, and these genetic variants affect the tumour cell, the microenvironment surrounding the tumour cell, or both. Moreover, depending upon the tumour type and situation, inflammatory networks of the immune system can play opposite roles, either promoting or inhibiting tumour susceptibility and progression.

In a football game, or any team, success is due to more than the sum of its parts, and even the fans have a big effect on the ultimate result. The fact of being vegan or eating raw food, for example, must have a relevance on Alien life, right? At the very least as much as the cheerleaders' optimism peps up the football team.

However, just when you think you've got it sorted, that you can instinctively influence this reality, there is always the statistical possibility that the reaction of so many thousands of genes will be different and that can bring you down again to a very physical world of pain. You have to remember not to let it do that, and not to be pulled back to the mathematical statistics.

Inspired by my sister's tales of bacteria, I try to keep flexible and to follow diverse rhythms. I am learning that, like marketing an artistic film, I need to think about how I sell these statistics to myself. You know, I would much rather have the four per

cent chance of surviving than the ninety-six per cent chance
of dying.

~

Three weeks into our stay, just as Bianca and I had established
a perfect routine in our beautiful neighbourhood, the gay
Italian-American owner knocked on our door and told us that
sadly he had found a new tenant who wanted to rent our
beautiful house for the whole year and give him proper money.
At the end of that week Bianca left for Paris, my mother came
to take over, and we moved to a little apartment near Chinatown.
Like any big American city, Washington DC has many faces,
but you only see the huge difference when you suddenly move
from the rich to the poor. And somehow, here it even seemed
as if the temperature had become colder.

I was delighted to embrace Margarita when she arrived back
from Macedonia, but I immediately sensed that she was
carrying with her the stress of the death of her father. Miro
had remained in Skopje with his now-widowed grandmother,
and without him that little apartment became the centre of
continuous discussions about everything. Too much bread, too
much meat, too little protein, more spicy, less sweet, every
detail of my life became the cause of an argument.*

Even in the best of times, my wife and my mother's person-
alities were prone to collide. I don't want to oversimplify a
complex family dynamic, but their two very different 'rhythms'
of life clearly had something to do with me often leaving the
apartment by myself. The tragicomic irony that kept running
through my head while I walked towards the multiplex cinema
in Chinatown was: I am living with an esteemed expert in
conflict resolution on one side of my house and a doctor trained

---

* Margarita: 'In Washington, the doctors had told me that, thanks to their work,
you might even survive for fourteen months. I asked them for something that could
calm me, to take the edge off. To which their reply was, "It is not part of this
protocol, we can't help you with this." And I could not cry with you. I could not
talk to you about any of this, because you were already somewhere else.'

in the most modern psychotherapy on the other side, and all they can do is argue and yell, without finding a peaceful compromise. And sadly, while walking back to our flat in the freezing cold, after watching two hours of full-on, superhero action and adventure, I don't think I felt any better, or calmer.

I remember getting up on a Saturday morning, walking out of our room and seeing my mother reading something. She smiled at me. 'How did you sleep?' I nodded my head to indicate 'OK' and she went on, 'You know, I went out early this morning, got a coffee at a Chinese shop, and found an Italian newspaper.'

At this point Margarita appeared in the living room and moved towards the kitchen area. My mother stood up and came towards us.

'I was thinking that we should talk to the doctors in Milan, and ask them what they think is the right therapy for you, so we can have a second opinion.'

As I made Margarita her coffee, she suddenly raised her voice, 'This is my breakfast . . . can you stop talking about this!'

My mother continued, 'In two weeks I am flying back, Margarita, and I have to make sure that we're doing the right thing. Perhaps you don't need to return to LA and we can all get a flight together back to Italy.'

Margarita, now with her cup of coffee in her hand, stormed towards our bedroom. 'You just can't stop with this constant attack, can you?' and slammed the door behind her. After a quiet minute, I walked towards our room, as the sound of her crying grew louder.

A week later, Margarita and I jumped on a low-budget bus and went for a weekend in New York, to be together in private. She had booked a lovely little hotel in midtown, where we finally felt calm together. The next morning, after having taken a shower, I brushed my hair and it started to fall off my head in clumps, a hole here and another elsewhere. I should have cut it all off at the beginning, but now I had to stick with these ridiculous gaps.

Fortunately it was winter, which allowed me to put on some hat or other and hide my dramatic hairstyle from the public. Margarita tried to cheer me up by lending me some of her creams, but there was nothing I could do. Looking at myself in the mirror, I realized that it was a very recognizable hairdo. I had never thought about it, but when you see a person with patches of hair fallen out, you understand immediately the background to that fashion statement.

While Margarita met her cousin, who was living there and working as a researcher, I went to meet the director of the Transcendental Meditation fund, whom Russell had introduced me to. I had talked with him a few times at Russell and Katy's wedding in India, and he seemed nice, but at that moment I had assumed he was simply one of Russell's new-age fads. Over the years he had dragged me into many similarly charming places, like the Hare Krishna church in London, where the people were very charming, but I had always been too pragmatic to allow such things to enter my already complex life. And I guess that is where I was wrong.

Even if this kind of world had been 'hippy shit' for me in the past, now, thanks to my Ned Flanders hypnotist, I was up for at least giving it a try. As he ate his bagel and told me stories about his job, I tried to spot the hippy side of this man, but I couldn't see any in him. He seemed like a classic New Yorker, a university professor, both calm and curious. He told me about the Transcendental Meditation teachers in DC and they sounded as normal as him. That evening I told Margarita about my new project with TM, and she seemed curious and excited, even more than I was, so I immediately booked us some meetings. It was perfect, something peaceful that we could do and explore together.

Just as spring started to show itself in Washington, we received some guests. It was really important for me that my

Uncle Antonio had flown in to pay us a visit. Bianca had organized a motel nearby, where he could stay with his younger boyfriend (only a year older than me) and Anna, his old high-school friend, who, at least in Siena during public events, acted as his beard. His boyfriend was very sweet and warm, and for me Anna had always been my aunt, or at least I treated her as such. Any woman who could deal with and accept Antonio's constant snappy remarks and comments was a saint, as far as I was concerned.

I had a weekend free from those machines, and as I stuck my head out of my bedroom window, I noticed that all the trees in DC had started to flower. With all the 'family' together, we walked around the lake in the centre of the city, passing statues of the presidents surrounded by cherry trees covered with white blossom – a gift from one of the Japanese emperors after the Second World War. It was stunning, and while we celebrated Antonio's seventy-first birthday in a big restaurant with a TV showing a football game, I had a feeling that perhaps my illness had started influencing my life positively and even helped me to embrace my family, for all its oddities.

Antonio had put together some funds from the family company and from one of my aunts. This help was absolutely crucial, as we had been living on every loan that we could get. He obviously complained of how poor he was now that the Italian economy was in a complete depression and the Sclavi bakery company was costing more to run than it was earning, but it was part of his character. He was not himself unless he was bickering and complaining about something, but right there, in that no-man's-land that is Washington DC, I started believing that we did share something, that his soul could not really be so far away from that of his brother, my father, who was generous in his very essence.

A week later, after I was finished with the trips in my Spaceship, I asked the doctors how it had all gone and was extremely disappointed to hear that they could not tell me very much. The images of the MRI had been completely obscured by the physical reaction of my brain cells to the radio bombs, and so I would have to wait for a few months before seeing any results. A few months, and then what?

I had come to the end of my current association with hospitals and doctors and frankly I did not know what I felt about it. All I had, as a reminder of their work with me, was a six-month meditative vacation before the next MRI, a big plastic bag full of cortisone – in case I felt pressure on my head – and some other boxes full of pills that everybody told me would prevent me from getting an epileptic seizure. A few docs had told me that it often happened to people who have had brain surgery. What a lovely reminder of our scientific liaison.

Margarita and I went back to LA, to meet up with different doctors and friends who might know of any new options. Russell, his bodyguard, Tom, Nicola and Nik were bouncing around the world promoting *Arthur*, which had just come out in cinemas in different parts of the world, so for at least a little while we could have 'our' old bedroom back. The supermarkets and streets of LA were covered by gigantic posters of Russell sitting cross-legged on a couch, smiling, surrounded by lovely, famous actresses. It was almost overwhelming to see his gigantic face everywhere.

I shaved off all the uneven hair that had been growing on the sides of my head, and kept the beard and top of my hair growing. The hope was not to scare Miro, who was about to arrive in LA with Jasmina, Margarita's mother. It wasn't completely clear why they were venturing on such a long and expensive trip. The only thing I knew was that Margarita really needed to have her boy with her right now. I had no idea how long we were going to stay in America, but perhaps taking Jasmina away from the city where she had lived with her husband since she was nineteen years old, could somehow also help her.

Now that we had both our child and a babysitter, we set up a double date with Amanda and Shepard Fairey to go and see *Arthur* together. We had first met them at Russell and Katy's wedding in India. The only things I knew about him then were that he had put his André the Giant graffiti street art on the walls in many cities where I had been, and he had become very famous with the Barack Obama 'HOPE' poster. Within minutes of meeting Shepard at the wedding, we were discussing art, politics and geography, and I knew immediately why Russell had wanted us to meet.

Throughout my illness in LA, our friendship had grown. We seemed to gel and understand each other on various levels, and as I sat there drinking a glass of sparkling water at the bar in the cinema, I realized that I had been missing this kind of conversation. I was delighted to see Margarita riff with his wife Amanda. She needed to get her head somewhere else, where cancer and death were not continuously centre stage.

The tales of my illness led us on to politics, which then brought us to art. Up to that moment I had not thought that art could be part of a therapy for me. It would be something I could control myself, without having to ask the opinion of three different doctors. I started thinking about how I could create art that would help my illness and how it would have to be social, and non-violent, and optimistic . . . and it would have to engage with that hole in my head. For one night at least, our minds were distracted from reality.

We sat down together and watched *Arthur*. It was a complex viewing in different ways and we all had mixed feelings. We liked it, and Russell was good in it, but . . . the film was a strange mix. It wanted to be sweet and emotional, while at the same time it had lots of crazy hilarious comedy set-ups in it. We had all tried to avoid reading the reviews before seeing the film, in order to give Russell our own impartial reviews.

In the end, a good part of the press reacted badly. People who knew the original film felt that their baby had been changed for the worse. From the beginning, the financiers knew that remaking a classic was going to be tricky, but no one could have predicted how intense the attacks would be.

Just a few months before, it seemed that Russell was going to be able to receive financing for just about anything he wanted. Now the game seemed to have flipped. The doors that were wide open before, now started to be closed by the film industry. While everyone continued to smile and be extremely friendly with Russell, there was an underlying feeling that, as soon as he walked out of the room, they would turn around and tell their staff to focus on other projects by someone who was hotter, younger or hipper.

This was not dissimilar to the sensation that stole over Margarita and me, as we walked away from our meetings with oncologists. I had done the brain operation and the radical radiotherapy, but now what? Why were we not being presented with new options?

I recall a particular afternoon, as I was sitting calmly in the garden outside our house, waiting for Margarita to come down, when I became aware that our need to live 'normally' and to look for houses or jobs, while also doing everything possible to keep me alive, must have seemed absurd to the world outside; but it was essential for my, or rather, *our* survival as a team.

This thread, of us living together but searching for parallel and discordant realities, is something that will continue throughout this tale. It took a little while for us to accept that we had no more buttons that we could push here and we were now forced to engage with a 'normal' life. But what did normal look like? Where was it?

We decided that going back home to Italy was perhaps not a bad idea and that we could enjoy a more modest and calm reality there. For me the priority was to find a new oncological outlook, where hopefully they would appreciate the first-class work that I had been doing on my brain here in America.

At the end of the day, returning to our house, to our self-made apartment and to Miro's play school, was going to do us all good, and who knows, it could even allow me to slowly detach myself from Margarita the doctor and re-find her as my wife.

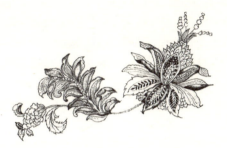

9

New Hope, New Life

Bologna, 2003

I am going to attempt to start this chapter by telling you about one of my favourite books, *The Name of the Rose*, by Umberto Eco, which is set in an Italian Abbey, where a Franciscan friar discovers that reading comedic verses is literally 'a deadly sin'. The book is tricky, in every way, as our author tells us in the introduction that it had been originally written by that monk in the fourteenth century and then translated into French in 1842, and along the way, it had got lost. And so we, as readers, are asked to believe in the memories of our author, which will become the one and only story.

In 2003 Umberto Eco was teaching semiotics in Bologna, where I had found financial and emotional refuge in the offices of Downtown Pictures – and where this chapter begins. All alone, like a little friar in that ancient town, I continued to think back to the rush of love that had passed through my veins for that Macedonian woman, for the first time in many years. I felt like an addict coming back to his dose after years of romantic celibacy. While rationally I should have cancelled all memories of that relationship, the attraction between Margarita and me was kept alive by my understanding of semiotics, which permitted me to stick to the alternative narrative voiced by my deeper emotions.

If this sentence sounds 'weird' to you, believe me, Alex's voice does not make it any clearer. But I am sure, if you think about it, you have your own romantic stories based on your emotional memories.

Bologna was exactly the right place in which to distract myself with the development of a series of fictional screenplays. Most days, in the huge office of Downtown Pictures, there was only me and Valentina Merli, a young woman who, like me, had worked abroad most of her life. Often at lunchtime we sat next to each other in the tiny restaurant next to our office, where the granddaughter of the matriarch chef would offer us different types of handmade pasta, and there we felt that we were somehow part of a backwards diaspora, carrying on our shoulders the necessary optimism to get Italy back on track.

As a good producer, Marco Muller had managed to sell us the idea of a necessary and exciting new future outside of Rome (where just about everything was happening). He is an impressive man, who speaks something like seven or eight languages. Listening to him as he talked on the phone, I got the impression that, from his time as director of the Locarno Film Festival, he had become fast friends with nearly every director in the world, from Hollywood box-office stars to Asian artists that I had never heard of.

Having won an Oscar the year before with *No Man's Land*, by the Bosnian director Danis Tanović, he had a realistic possibility of producing innovative films. As he often explained to the newspapers, his new company was not going to be in competition with anyone, as he would only be producing films from directors that none of the rival companies seemed to even notice.

Within a few weeks I was featured with Valentina and an assistant from Bologna (a lovely person whose name has been cancelled from my head) in a photo in the local newspaper. We represented hope and renewal for the whole town, and particularly for the younger, creative generation. Our energy was great and I was eager to finally succeed.

We had a whole bunch of projects in development with some great Italian and international documentary makers, comic-book authors, photographers, theatre writers and directors. It seemed incredible that this talent was all over the country but no one, apart from us, wanted to believe and invest in it.

There was a German director who was making a documentary about a group of priests who live on top of a mountain and never speak. An Italian director who planned to give a fresh look at life in the town of Pompeii a few days before Vesuvius erupted and burned it all away. They were all beautiful projects, but because they were 'art house' films, if the TV stations did not accept them, they had to be dropped. Unfortunately, it was often my responsibility to pass on this crushing information to our directors, who had placed their dreams on our seemingly sturdy shoulders.

Marco liked me because the work I did with Emily was brave, intellectually stimulating and fun, but I quickly realized that, in the world of art house, it is difficult to use the word 'fun' or 'funny'. In any case, I had a job. It was not very much money, but I had a proper contract that ensured I received a monthly wage. I could sit down with grumpy people like my Uncle Antonio in Siena and hold my head high. I had never made it my priority, but I could learn to appreciate the idea of a steady life in one location – and why not Bologna?

When going to Rome for meetings with Rai television or other financiers, I usually took a ride with Marco Muller and then crashed on a couch with my old friend Matteo, or his brother Blasco. The company did not have money for hotel rooms, but as a perk from our boss's many friends, I could get to see almost every theatre and dance show in town. One day I received a text from Margarita telling me that she was going to the theatre to see a modern dance show. It took me a few minutes to realize that, not only was it the first time I had heard from her since our last evening with the three bottles of wine, but without even thinking about it, my fingers had moved up and down instinctively, and had already replied.

I had arrived in Rome only the day before, which I guess could have been a simple coincidence, but during a meeting that day, I had also been given a ticket to that very same show. I don't know if I had ever been to a modern dance performance before, and the likelihood that on my first time there I was going to meet Margarita was, well, let's call it simply a *startling* coincidence.

I stood outside the theatre smoking a cigarette and talking to Rosanna – Matteo and Blasco's mother – who had a season ticket for all these kinds of shows. As Margarita arrived, I introduced her to Rosanna, struggling to find the right words to explain our 'friendship' to her. Fortunately we heard a ringing bell which forced us to walk in. I asked Margarita to follow me, knowing that the ticket I had from Muller's contact was in the Royal Box. There was a free seat right next to me, so even if we didn't have a chance to talk, we ended up watching the show sitting next to each other, with our bodies almost touching.

It was fantastic. The dancers were great, but the thing that really stuck in my mind was that one of them had no legs, zero, nothing, and just did the whole show moving his body freely with his arms and hands. Later we walked quietly out through the crowd together, as if neither of us wanted to break the spell. As soon as we met Rosanna outside on the street, we told her, almost finishing each other's sentences, every little detail that we loved. Feeling embarrassed, we continued talking without looking each other in the eye, aware that the other probably had an even bigger smile on their face. As I was staying at Matteo's apartment in Rosanna's house, I said goodbye to Margarita and left. It wasn't possible that I had made peace with her through that dance show. Was it?

The week after, I was off to Sicily in search of a location for the next film by the Hungarian master Béla Tarr. Muller introduced most of our future directors to us as 'the master', and since I had never heard of them or their work, I simply accepted that, in their own countries at least, they must have done something important. Béla Tarr had acquired the rights for the Georges Simenon story, *The Man from London*, and needed me to help him find a seaside town with a port. He had already gone around most of Europe looking for the perfect location, and had a premonition that he would find it in Sicily.

While I drove him and his lovely German assistant through Sicily, Béla explained to me what he was looking for. In the mid-2000s, getting a tape copy of one of his films was not easy, so embarrassingly I had never seen anything he had done. From what I had heard from Muller, most of his films were in black and white, and his most famous project, *Werckmeister Harmonies*, was over seven hours long, with two intermissions. What I did not know was that I was about to enter a parallel reality of cinematography, where each single day I would learn more than I would in a whole year in any film school.

With a constant cigarette parked in his mouth, and a grumpy tone of voice, Béla fit perfectly the stereotype of the old-school, East European director. When I asked him in what century the story was going to be set, he replied, 'No time. These are characters who have existed and will always exist.'

What he needed for his film was simply Béla world and Béla time, which I was now eager to learn and measure. From what I understood, his camera movements were the narrators of the story. In most normal films, the camera cuts away several times during a scene, from one character to the other, from one perspective to another. For Béla, the camera never stops filming until the scene is finished. If his camera needs eight minutes, his crew have to find, or create, a world that will fit it. The way he said it was, 'Most modern films are built on: Information, cut, Information, cut. Just to move the story along.'

I obviously looked confused, so he told me, 'I try to involve in my film other parts of life that are not necessarily concerning story movement. You should not be connecting directly with the story in a way that it looks like a chain. We pay the Simenon family good money for the story, but the story is not so important. You don't need to know the Why. You should feel the human relations. And not necessarily consciously.'

Enjoyable as our trip round Sicily had been, we didn't find a place that corresponded with Béla's vision for his film. After I returned to Bologna, Margarita and I started to communicate casually until, at some point, she offered to take a train and come up north to visit me. I was anxious about my emotions for her. I could not read them, even less manage them, and that was unfamiliar territory for me, to say the least.

Margarita came and we talked through all our dreams and interests, while she admired my pasta with fish (which I only made for special occasions); and although driven by very strong emotions, I managed, at least for that first night, to make her sleep on a couch in the living room.

We knew that we were on fragile ground – we weren't living in the same city and her study visa was going to expire in a couple of months – but I guess we had to let the passage of time decide for us. When I took Margarita to the train station, we looked at each other and kissed, and so resolved that this time we would not let our emotions slip away.

I liked and felt united with the other people there in Bologna, who were working with me to try and make this production company work. Muller's approach to culture and production was extremely exciting for me, but I was also worried that our start-up funds were being depleted and nothing substantial was coming back our way. In the beginning, Marco used to stop by as he walked through our office and tell us some amusing tales from his trips and meetings, but now his comments were infused with bitterness and were primarily focused on our failures.

One day, Muller's lovely assistant asked me if I had been telling people that I was no longer going to be with the company. The concept had never entered my head, so I was a bit puzzled. She went next door, spoke with Muller, and forced us to go out and take a cup of coffee together. I found out I was going to be laid off at the end of the summer.

Margarita had originally arrived in Italy intending to stay for only six months, but now that she had managed to prolong her stay and her friend, who shared the double bed with her, had gone back to Macedonia, the other half of that bed was . . . empty. The manager of her hotel-apartment near the main train station was very nice and had allowed Margarita to stay, and pay only her half of the weekly rent. Even if paying for the other half of that bed was not financially feasible for me, there was absolutely no way that as soon as I arrived in Rome I was not going to be sleeping next to her. So, all my entrances and exits of that room had to be . . . engineered.

I went about Rome looking for film companies who might employ me and found that no one needed my international experience. My parents' friends had explicitly warned me not to come back to Italy, as it would never compare to the experiences I'd had while living abroad, but I wasn't going to give up. I just needed to find a job that would keep me as close as possible to Margarita.

A few weeks later, while sitting in her little room, I received a call from Béla Tarr himself. He had been calling Muller and never getting an answer. After I'd told him that I was no longer working at Downtown Pictures, but most probably the channels weren't accepting his project, he said goodbye and hung up.

A few minutes later, just as I was telling Margarita about how cool I found Béla, he called me back and told me that he had found his location in France, in the city of Bastia on the island of Corsica, and offered me a job line-producing his *The Man from London*.

I started my back-and-forth meetings between Budapest and Corsica, and every day I worked with Béla's producer, trying to be creative with their very optimistic budget. The financing was pasted together with little bits of public funding from many countries and investors, and from the very beginning it felt like we were riding a small boat in a big stormy ocean.

I now understood that Béla's films could easily take a few years to shoot and I was going to have several months of hiatus every year. While his Hungarian crew were used to it, I was trying to get my head around how to live like this. Firstly, I needed to earn enough money to pay for a proper apartment where Margarita and I could live, and secondly, I could not imagine her waiting for me in Rome for six months of the year, while I hung out with a bunch of Hungarian dudes in a cold French port.

I had spent all my life travelling, and I believed that was the primary reason why I had not managed to have a true, lasting emotional relationship with anyone. Béla's world was exciting, but no matter how cool his director of photography was, for the first time in many years I was going to prioritize my romantic relationship over the needs of my artists. Yes, I had an addiction to a job that excited and stimulated me every day, but I now found myself dependent on a woman who was not associated with my job, and whose creativity I needed to manage in a completely different way.

I was in love.

Rome, London, Siena, 2004

There's a little park on one of the seven hills, where I had shot a scene for a German short film, which is by far the most romantic place in Rome. It's . . . Villa . . . something, I've forgotten. When I came back to Rome for summer holidays as a teenager, I used to go up there to get stoned with my friends; every tree bears gigantic oranges and the view is simply spectacular. You see everything from . . . aah, forget it, I'm just never going to remember any of those names. Why are some of the verbs still in my brain, yet I can't find most nouns?

The important part that I haven't forgotten, though, is that in that spring I took Margarita up there, and as we sat with our legs entwined on the edge of the railing, I looked at her and told her, 'You are my foundation, you give me excitement every day, and for that . . .', waving my arm across that fantastic view, 'I thank this city for having brought us together. You know that I'll always have to do some travelling, but—'

Margarita interrupted, hugging me fiercely, 'And I'll be there, travelling with you.'

'You would even come to Germany with me?'

'At school I was forced to learn German. I just never used it.'

After a long kiss, I continued, 'You know that it can be quite cold up in Berlin, and you are a warm-water fish . . .'

Before I could come to the end of that sentence, she looked at me as if I doubted her, and said quickly, 'We'll spend winter here, and during spring, once in a while, you can work up there.' We stared into each other's eyes, then she surprised me with '*Ich liebe dich*' and a kiss.

A week later, I flew to London, but before throwing myself

into the hectic life of that great city, I had to do a little stop on the way. I had organized for my darling friend (*name to be remembered, please, brain*), Russell's costume designer from his MTV show, to give me a ride to a town nearby (*maybe Bury St Edmunds?*) where Russell had been living clean for a month. I knew that he was only allowed to leave that place for a few hours a week, and as I arrived, it felt as if I was picking him up from a high security prison.

We walked out of there and I put my hands on his shoulders in a brotherly gesture, and it felt as if his body was weak and drained. The sensation almost scared me, but as our eyes met, I understood that he was completely clean. He had finally signed off the divorce papers with Heroine. Together with Mr Gee, a poet that he had recently met, we stopped off in a coffee shop in the main square.

He explained to me that in order to come out of addiction, he had to go through a process that was a million miles away from what we had tried to do. He told me that he now had to look at himself as an addict, who had created harm to himself and to others around him, and that his illness was always going to be with him. From now on his priority was to keep his addiction in check, which meant that he was going to attend Alcoholics Anonymous meetings for the rest of his life. The fact that AA was going to be his priority did not necessarily exclude his secondary addictions to fame and large-breasted women. He just had to make sure that the latter would not make him fall back into his former relationships.

As he finished telling me about his new life, his smile came back, the rhythm of his voice lifted, and I realized that I hadn't stopped laughing for several minutes. I found myself taking a deep breath – his comic timing was still there.

I could see that even if they took away his drugs, all his tricks and toys, and even his ego, no one would ever take away his wit. We walked back to the Focus 12 rehab centre, where other addicts were out in the garden smoking cigarettes, and I gave

Russell a hug then left to catch my bus to London. I knew that he had finally found a place that could truly help him.

The first stop on my London trip was with an old German friend. George Lenz is an extremely charming man, who has always shown an interest in my projects. He would come to Brixton when I was a bartender, and while I tried to show off my talent with my creative cocktails, he would tell me of the films in which he was acting and the new energy that was pulsing through German cinema. We kept in touch and somehow always managed to meet in extraordinary bars. From Bologna to Salzburg to Berlin, our wine-infused discussion of the prospect for European film never finished.

A few years before he had introduced me to the film director George Milton, with whom he had shared many adventures, amongst which was a feature film called *Appetite*. Both Georges are the children of creative fathers with big egos. While Milton grew up on tour with his father's conceptual puppet-theatre act, Lenz followed his father's love affair with the German post-war Zero art movement. Having been raised with art, they shared a belief in making sophisticated popular films.

That evening, Lenz took us out in London to one of his favourite restaurants and made us drink various superlative wines until the three of us, drunk as skunks, crashed in his hotel bed together, swearing to each other that we would create a company that would revolutionize European cinema. And so it was that the German, British, Italian company '2 Many Executives' was born. The European Union was obviously going to be the future and with that brave statement of intent, I felt sure the world would quickly embrace us.

Milton and his co-writer Mark Tilton had a screenplay called *The Truth* that they had developed a few years ago for Channel 4's film division, which I believed was perfect for our first production, as it was set in a single location and we could make it for a low budget without waiting years for financing. We could start casting that sophisticated British comedy, while

I would look for other similarly inventive, trans-national tales throughout Europe.

My search for Italian authors was exciting in so many ways, and it also legitimized my renting an apartment with Margarita in Rome. As we carried our suitcases up to the third floor and arrived in our new apartment, almost inside the Vatican, we smiled at each other in elation, and kissed.

I don't know if you have ever seen the Vatican, or what opinion you might hold towards the Catholic Church, but to this day I still feel like a child walking through Disneyland every time I pass by there. But in contrast to its American wonderland version, the energy that I felt during that period when we would stroll down those streets hand in hand was undoubtedly real. We would walk from our apartment and not even notice the constant flocks of tourists that were everywhere with their maps, books and guides.

While Margarita was working at the Policlinico hospital, I went around Rome in search of scripts and writers who could develop stories that my friend Matteo and I could put in for state financing. While Matteo had worked in the legal side of production in Italy, through my time with Marco Muller I had got to know many of the younger directors and authors. Once again I was not going to have much money, but my hopes were high.

Throughout our relationship I had always tried to explain to Margarita the social dynamics of making films. We quickly take our own world for granted, and only realize how unusual it is when someone from the outside makes us notice it. For example, if you grew up in a socialist country, where everyone had a fixed job that would always finish at four in the afternoon, to allow them to meet up with friends or grow vegetables in their garden or dacha, you might find the erratic rhythms of my own profession slightly disturbing.

The rhythm in which a film is being shot can bring stress even to the best relationships. While on a daily schedule, a couple can find their rhythm: 'When are you back home? Can you do the shopping?' While shooting a film, you end up putting 120 per cent of your energy and emotion into the film, and your partner inevitably starts to see your job as your lover, taking priority over everything else in your life.

They can call you while you are on set and you reply, 'You have a bad cold? I'll talk to you later. Right now I'm in a night shoot in the middle of a difficult scene. Love you.' The inescapable thought is, what are you doing with all those handsome actors and actresses at night? For a whole week? For a whole month? You can't help it. I knew that Margarita – and I will always love her for that – was not a jealous person, and so we would somehow make our relationship work. The other and much more complex issue was that, whilst I had grown up in a family where my parents were more united then ever when they were apart, Margarita, having grown up as a single child, had a strong aversion to being left alone, and I couldn't do very much about that.

While waiting for the Italian state financing, I focused on the UK, where *The Truth* was almost ready to go. The basic story of *The Truth* that got our fantastic cast excited was this: 'Seven strangers go to a remote retreat for a week of soul-searching. Encouraged to tell the truth at all times by their guru Donna Shuck, they venture on a spiritual journey of personal growth, taking in jealousy, hatred, sex, perversion and a little murder on the way.'

After I had been away filming our first film on location for over a month, our love grew even stronger. We would go to parties and events and not even think of talking to other people. On one such evening, Anna Negri, the birthday girl, approached us and said jokingly, 'This is *my* party, and you can't come here and exclude me from it. You'll make everybody here jealous!'

We had to leave our apartment near the Vatican, and through some other friends found a tiny three-storey house near the Coliseum. It was the most romantic little house imaginable.

While Margarita painted flowers on paper and stuck them to the walls, on every trip to London I would bring back Indian fabrics, which we used to cover all the walls of our living room.

There was no time for ifs, ands or buts. The time was right. The time was now. We went to the beach and while splashing in the water I knelt down and there, submerged in the Tyrrhenian Sea, I found her hand and put a ring on it.

I spent a considerable amount of time cutting and pasting photographs into a romantic book of our relationship, and on the last page, I humbly asked Margarita's parents for their daughter's hand in marriage. I sent it off and was quite proud of my presentation until, a few weeks later, the postman arrived with a large box containing a set of stunningly designed, handcrafted paintings and a beautifully written text in Macedonian.

Her parents were from a different culture. Their emotions, like Margarita's, were expressed ten times louder than anyone I had ever met before. I know that in America or the UK I often appear eccentric when I hug and kiss everyone. It is a normal part of Italian communication, like saying 'Ciao' both at the beginning and the end of a meeting, but Macedonians find this insufficient and insist on giving three kisses upon meeting, and that applies for all men and women.

Our first wedding was in January, in Rome's town hall. I call it the first wedding because, although it was a beautiful private event, it was going to be followed by a bigger celebration in the summer for our families and friends, who were all in different parts of the world. My Uncle Antonio had offered us the use of Villa Flora for our special occasion.

On my next trip to London I went to visit Russell, who was clean as a whistle and had more energy than a teenage monkey. We sat outside his posh new house in Hampstead, drinking tea and smoking cigarettes. As he told me about his experiences shooting a big American film in Hawaii, and the general excitement for him out there, I told him how, while swimming in the sea with Margarita, I had bent down and almost drowned asking her to marry me.

That was one of the few times I have seen him freeze up. Russell Brand, nothing to say? A mate of his was really tying the knot. Constantly, forever and ever the same person. For better, for worse and all that stuff. A reality that I knew had not yet hit him. He had seen the development of my relationship with Margarita, but was surprised nevertheless. Finally, his reply was, 'Marriage? That is a big commitment.'

We laughed and I asked him if he could take over the role of the priest for our wedding. I knew that amongst the various characters that lived in his strange brain, between his rendition of the Elephant Man and the Man Pissing His Pants, Russell had always cherished the idea of being a Messiah, or at the very least, a priest. In fact, I think it was the first and only time I have seen him properly excited to have been cast for a role. (I must admit that five years after my wedding, when he told me that he wanted to marry Katy Perry, I did have a similar reaction.)

The date of our wedding was 4 July, which happened to be Russell's birthday – his thirtieth birthday. He arrived in Tuscany with his mother Babs and his girlfriend at the time. He came to my uncle's country house in Siena and, with his most professional attitude, walked through all the rooms where people were arranging the different aspects of the event, and learned the name and role of each member of both families. By the end of the day, he had charmed all our relatives and helped me to decide the last details of our wedding ceremony with its mixture of Macedonian and Italian traditions.

When I casually asked him what was going to be his attire as our priest, he told me that he had decided to wear white. Many people, including me, had told him that you don't wear white at a wedding unless you are getting married, but I knew him well enough to understand that when he makes a decision, he sticks to it. Margarita and I laughed, because we knew that by putting such different cultures so tightly together we had already created plenty of potential for humour, and his entrance in white was going to be the cherry on top for the more traditional members of my family.

Margarita and I had gone together to buy her wedding dress, and I knew that her crew of Macedonian and Serb friends would be stitching and re-stitching it until the very last second. I had been to a few weddings in Yugoslavia and knew that it might become a bit bizarre for some of my guests, but fortunately Matteo, who was my best man, had come to the event dressed as an Indian guru, which gave a direct sign to the guests that the whole day was going to be . . . unusual. He helped me to galvanize our friends, who were more than glad to take apart the traditional idea of groomsmen or ushers, to embrace this folkloristic game.

They picked up drums, whistles and other instruments and accompanied me to stand below the little terrace of Villa Flora, where I was supposed to entice the bridesmaids to show me my future wife. As is their tradition, we tried to sing her songs, dance and yell in unison until the girls, accompanying her, brought her out for me to see. The maids of honour interrupted the applause and told me that Margarita was precious and that I would have to give them a lot of money to take her away from them. My whole team and all the guests laughed, but it was not actually a joke.

I threw all the coins I could find up there, until they finally agreed to bring her down the stairs, but as I got close to her, the maids of honour told me to take off her shoe and put some money in it. I put some in and the girls all yelled, 'How cheap! You can't get her for that!' I put in some more money, and at this point I had started to drop in twenty-Euro notes, but as Margarita tried to step into her shoe, she glanced back at her friends, who looked very sad. They couldn't believe that their lovely and beautiful friend was going to live with such a poor man.

This continued until I had put in everything that I had in my wallet and even some more that I had borrowed from my mates. When Margarita eventually pressed her naked foot into her shoe, full of fifty- and twenty-Euro notes, and turned back to her friends with a smile, they stepped away from her and told me they were satisfied, and I could finally kiss the bride.

Russell had got thoroughly into his priest role, and led the whole audience through every step of the ritual. As my father was no longer with us, we had decided that it would be the two mothers who would give the speeches towards the end of the ceremony. The day before, a bit anxious, I had asked my mother what she was going to read at our wedding. She started reciting me one of her favourite poems by Martin Niemöller, 'First they came for the Socialists . . . Then they came for the Jews, and I did not speak out – Because I was not a Jew . . .'

I was visibly shocked and raised my hand to pause her, and in my most diplomatic tone of voice, I said, 'Mum, let's think about this for a second. This is really not the most romantic contribution that you can bring to a wedding. Do you realize that?' She thought about it for a few seconds and said, 'OK, fine, I am sure that I have a version of the *Divine Comedy* in my room.'

So fortunately, on the day, she ended up reciting a piece of Dante's *Inferno* (the one about Paolo and Francesca's love, in the fifth song), which many of my Italian friends knew by heart and recited with her.

When the applause for my mother's poem ended, Margarita's mother Jasmina stepped into centre stage right underneath us, and without any book or paper in her hands, gazed straight at us and started reciting a poem in Macedonian, which was a mesh of pure emotions. Even if I didn't understand her language, somehow, looking at her eyes filling with tears, and following the rise and fall of her voice expressing love, pride and good wishes, I was kept spellbound – along with everyone else.

To bring us back to a more familiar emotional reality, Russell recited one of his favourite passages from Shakespeare and then explained to the whole audience that according to the Macedonian tradition, at this stage the two mothers needed to put their hands on a large ritual cake and split it in two. The symbolism of this being, as Russell explained to the audience, 'whoever gets the biggest piece, their child will rule the relationship'. A moment of tension and then . . . *Crack!* . . . Jasmina was holding ninety per cent of the cake, which left my mother with a little lonesome piece in her hands.

If it had been a film, we would have started hearing the wind pick up, and followed the bouncing little crumbs that had fallen from that precious cake, all the way along the floor until they stopped abruptly at Margarita's shoe, full of money. Breaking the silence that ensued, Russell exclaimed, 'They are perfectly equal parts! They will rule their family together!' And so, in some way, saving my honour.

We all walked up to the dining area of the gardens, where Margarita and I started the dance with Dean Martin's classic, 'When the moon hits your eye like a big pizza pie . . . That's amore,' breaking up the intense emotions of the sacred ritual. During the lunch there was a continuous Macedonian dance going on, where a long row of people held each other's hands and simultaneously took three steps right, and then one back. After a visit from the gypsy band, Margarita's father Stojan sat down at the piano and played us some traditional tunes with a few of his friends, and so it continued until nightfall, when the classic songs were replaced by modern dance tunes, mixed by Umberto, an old friend from Bologna.

One great bonus of getting married was that our families had decided to put some of their savings together and help us purchase an apartment of our own in Rome. In 2005 the real-estate market was booming and everyone believed it would continue in this direction for many years to come. After quickly realizing that we were not going to find our dream house anywhere near the centre of Rome, we started exploring parts of the city where we had never been. I had heard from many friends that Pigneto, a neighbourhood not far from the main train station, was going to become the next hip, cool part of town.

In our first exploration of the area, Margarita and I found an apartment with a huge roof terrace which, with our family's money and a mortgage, could become ours. The fact that it needed to be completely reconstructed made us all the more excited. With the assistance of Jasmina, who is an architecture professor in Skopje, we would finally be able to express our love by shaping together every part of *our* house.

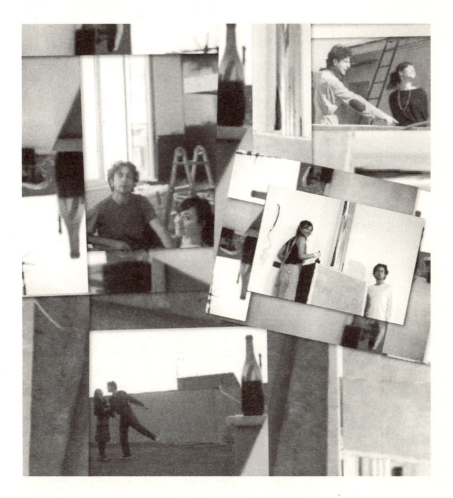

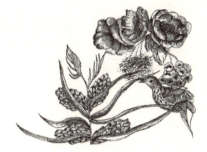

10

Oncological Gonzo Journalism

*Note: this is when I actually started writing. I set up a
'Friends' email group and started sending them regular
news of what was happening in Italy, and as the various
bits of feedback came my way, I realized that this type
of communication was absolutely essential for my survival.*

Rome, 2011

God, I am sure you will not mind if, in my hour of need, I
start getting involved with one of your many belief systems.

There are so many options, so many possibilities, and I really can't lay my faith wholly on these doctors; I have to balance their hypotheses with something else, something stronger. You are good at blessing things, so let's start with Transcendental Meditation, and while you are there, let's also bless the CD that the hypnotist gave me in DC, as my day-to-day reality would not be possible without them. I also need to add the smile of my son in the morning, because it is just as important to my good health as any of these theories that people are bouncing into my brain.

Living in what was undeniably the best research centre in the world was extremely calming. While I was at the NIH in Bethesda, Maryland, I was constantly surrounded by the truth that lies in science, and I felt as if everyone was focused on discovering a cure for my illness. The American attitude, with which I was also partly raised, reminded me continuously that, 'I am the best! And No Matter What . . . I will WIN this battle!'

Now, sitting in a bar in lovely Rome, where tourists from all over the world walk by and snap endless pictures for sharing on social media, no one takes any notice of me. The language is different, but so what? It is my mother tongue, which I speak naturally. I know instinctively how to move my hands to communicate surprise, hatred, disinterest or lack of responsibility. If it is such a familiar world, why can I not make sense of anything that is happening here? And let's not start with Italian politics . . . let's just put it in a box for the time being, as I have some other issues to resolve.

In this land of countless churches, none of the people I meet seem to believe in the same thing. Everyone has a radical opinion about what I should do, which makes my belief in science problematic. The basic concept of science is that the theories should be falsifiable. Going to meet doctors and neurosurgeons can't be like a discussion with a bunch of people in a bar, where everyone has a different opinion about what happened last Sunday at the game that took place in my brain between Aliens and good bacteria.

While one doctor here in Rome says, 'I don't think you have a chance with that radiotherapy. It won't do anything for you,' the other one criticizes the work of Dr Vogel in America, saying, 'It's bullshit. All of it. They didn't actually cut anything away.' One of the few things that has been reiterated by different doctors is that the surgery has taken out a maximum of ten per cent of the cancer in my brain, while there in LA land, they spoke of seventy or eighty per cent. *What?* And what about all the work that I did in Washington DC with the super machines – did that not really achieve anything, either?

The Romans say that it is all unclear because of that radiotherapy – but if I wait six months for it to calm down, the Aliens will have already grown to parts of my brain where no one can operate. Since I have spent five days a week, for a month and a half, with the most sophisticated radiology computer in the world, how can it be that the results are a simple matter of opinion? With my hands clutching the top of my head in desperation, the Italian words that force themselves out of my mouth . . . well, let's just say they cannot be written, especially since these days I have to be very pure, as I'm calling on all the spiritual beings I've ever met.

I've become addicted to meditation because of Russell's relationship with the film director David Lynch, which does not necessarily give it a legitimacy in the oncology departments of Italy; but as each one of those first-rate scientists seems to be following their own religion, and all of them feel like science fiction, I can certainly put some of my trust in the man who brought me *Twin Peaks* and *Mulholland Drive*.

God, I know you have a sense of humour, and thank you for having helped me surround my life with comedy, but please, please, at least at this stage, can we get serious? The doctors are talking about chopping out pieces of my brain, and maybe (and let's keep it at maybe now) that I'll even being awake when it happens.

I'll meditate and go to sleep, hopefully not thinking of *Wild at Heart*. There are enough crazy creatures in my brain already, and I don't think I could take that one as well.

~

Today, I went to Rome's Policlinico hospital to do one more round of doctor visits. The primary issue that I'm trying to resolve before August, when everyone is off on holiday, is: do I need to have an operation to remove the remainder of the tumour in my brain before the summer break? And there are multiple subsidiary issues. Is there a problem if I don't do it now? What are the risks? Should I do it awake? Is it safer awake, even though it does sound scarier? The list of questions seems endless, as does the variety of answers given to me by the different doctors.

Margarita's best woman at our civil wedding here in Rome was Dottoressa Ada Francia. I'm telling you that because she's the top Professor of Neurology in the Policlinico hospital and so has access to all the neurosurgeons, which makes her my most crucial guide in this mad world.

Neurosurgeons are Hollywood stars in the world of doctors, and perhaps even outside it. They become famous for having performed dangerous operations that no one else would ever attempt, and nobody here talks about operations having gone badly, which I guess is good news for me.

Today we went to Ada Francia's office, where she told us about the various neurosurgeons that we should meet. She looks at the world in three or four layers, and that's probably why she's so successful in the flora and fauna of doctors' egos. Ada always has an opinion about everything, but in this particular case she remains silent on her choice of the best surgeon, and I understand this is one of those leaps that I will have to make alone.

Fortunately, Ada has set up a bunch of meetings for Margarita and me to get to know my potential neurosurgeons. I must say that casting actors for this conceptual art performance in my brain is difficult. Margarita and I went to meet two of the top docs today and as both of them made us wait in their dark, narrow hallway for over half an hour, I realized that they have a certain way of moving around the hospital that clearly communicates: 'Leave me alone, don't speak to me.'

Both were small men, and both walked into their offices and closed the doors behind them, without even faintly acknowledging the presence of the people waiting for them outside. For me, the most stressful amount of time ended up being those eight minutes when the first surgeon was in there all alone, surely aware of how high my stakes were. Tom Waits' song floated into my mind: 'What's he building in there?'

I waited in that dark hallway in the Policlinico, hoping that we would find someone who truly inspired us, and could make us both feel at ease with the impending operation. I smiled at Margarita, lowering my hand in a sign of disappointment at the doctors' tiny stature, and she covered her mouth, trying to hold back her laughter. I am tall, and I don't want a little hobbit to cut my brain apart.

While waiting there, I imagined someone like Vin Diesel in *Pitch Black* appearing, or Russell Crowe in *Gladiator*. One of my favourites is Nicolas Cage, but I am not sure if I would cast him. I am afraid he might start flipping out during the operation. No, no, no. I must choose some professorial-type man, who works the land in his spare time. His hands have to be as steady as a rock and as soft as silk. Whoever I choose . . . be careful! Please.

~

After interminable discussions with different and extremely highly qualified doctors, with full control of a medical vocabulary that is (I assume) explicitly designed to exclude normal humans from the conversation, I can confirm that the words 'unequivocal' or 'certain' are not to be adopted in my personal medical lexicon. There will always be another doctor with a very convincing and opposite theory.

This medical debate has had long and complex repercussions on my relationship with my wife in the past months. When we sit down with these doctors, and before I even say a word, I notice that their eyes focus only on Margarita. They know that she was Ada's student and so will actually understand their jargon. In our relationship, as it developed from the beginning, I was the one who mediated her battle against the Italian legal system that wanted to kick her out of the country because she was an immigrant. I was the one that continuously fought for her in this extremely masculine culture.

But now the roles have been completely reversed and she is the one that is fluent in their language, and who after every meeting has to translate it to me in a vocabulary that I can understand.* I love her for trying to teach me the importance of their semantics, but I don't seem to have the time or patience for it. It feels like those discussions between political parties in parliament. You can talk your way into anything, but at some point, someone has to stand up and say, 'Are we going to cut these aliens away or not?'

Not for the first time, one of Antonio Gramsci's quotes saved me: 'The point of modernity is to live a life without illusions while not becoming disillusioned.'

~

I've made up my mind. Many of the technical discussions were resolved in the end by choosing the neurosurgeon that I simply like and trust the most on a human level. It is Professor Santoro: the old-school doctor, the head of the department, whom Ada in her silence seemed to trust the most. He is the one who

---

* Margarita: 'Once I came back to Italy, I stepped into the role of being the one who has to save your life. The healer. I had to just find the doctors and organize that other part and those people.'

appears to have the least dogmatic approach. While talking with some of the others, I had the sensation that they were too eager to get this job. Maybe it was only my imagination, but I felt as if they were trying to sell me something that I simply could not swallow.

My man has clocked off more operations than anyone else there. When I met him today, I asked him again about the surgery without general anaesthetic, and looking straight into my eyes, he managed to calm me down. It is probable that he will do it while I am conscious, but he will make that call when we are closer to the operation. If someone can sell you the idea that being awake while getting your brain cut is cool, he must be a magician. In any case, the results of his decision will only be seen once the operation has been done, and my brain has become a bit lighter. I dreamed of that operation last night, and I hope that his calm and steady eyes will help me sleep better from now on.

~

Today I heard that the stars have realigned and I will be operated on before the August break. This is public health, so nothing is straightforward, and I'm sure that Margarita's connections will be essential for finding me an empty bed in the neurosurgery department, from where I will then be shifted to a different room to prepare for surgery. I'm getting ready for a radically different experience than the Kaiser Permanente where I ended up in LA, and where the luxury of the private room with a view of the Scientology headquarters cannot be equalled.

If everything else is stable at the end of this week, I shall be called to occupy a bed in the hospital and start running a round of tests that will prepare me for an operation around 25 July. This is all theory until it happens, but the will is there. Mostly I trust the doctors and will feel comfortable with them carving up my brain. Well . . . as comfortable as one can be with that concept. The rest is keeping cool, meditating, keeping the family cool as well, and going for the experience of it. Obviously . . . One day at a time.

~

Because I am not officially an urgent case, nor in imminent clinical risk, neither Ada nor the neurologist can get me a bed in the department. The reason is that in a country that would like to pride itself on its welfare state, the free beds in the neurosurgical ward should be given to the people who have the clearest 'need' and not the ones who have the larger amount of money. That is all true and I agree, but I have been told by the big professor that in a week or so I will be having an operation. How do I do that if I can't get in the door?

Although checking into the hospital by way of A & E doesn't make sense to me right now, I am told it's the only way I can do this. Breaking and entering into the state clinic wasn't going to be an easy feat and it took some planning and co-ordination between the team. The general idea was that, once I got in there, we would alert our contacts and as soon as a bed was free, they would transfer me to the second floor where my big doc hangs out.

As I skimmed through the newspapers this morning, I realized that they are full of stories about the imminent collapse of the economy. It seems that we'll know if the world economy is really on the brink of collapse around the date of my operation. It could be that I will be offering my brain to medical exploration exactly when President Obama is delivering his speech on the 2nd or 3rd of August. Maybe when I wake up from surgery, I'll find that a new economic system has exploded upon the world – or maybe my vision will have changed radically due to the surgery and I will never know the truth and I will assume that everything is just hunky dory.

~

A & E is the only truly humane medical institution of any country. The only place where, if you are ill, they will not ask you for money or your insurance; their basic principle is to cure you (or at least within the terms of the emergency). As had happened to me on that miraculous day in LA.

If you have some illness, A & E can't refuse you, and explaining to the world that I have an illness is not one of the problems I have had in the last six months. What I had not considered is that A & E also cannot deny assistance to all the junkies and alcoholics who want to take a break, or simply get off the street for a few days. Smacked-out, transsexual prostitutes needing cures before going back to work, delirious senior citizens whose family want to park them somewhere for the holidays – all of those can't be refused from A & E either. They are sick, just like I am.

While preparing to break into A & E, I was too self-involved to understand the reality that I would have to confront in there. After all, the advice had been, 'Arrive at A & E exaggerating your symptoms slightly and, as soon as we have a bed free, we'll take you up to our department. Maximum in one day.'

I played my part of the ill man, with Margarita proving herself much better at presenting my case as an emergency than I did, and it all worked smoothly. Without any waiting time, I was placed on one of the beds in A & E. What the neurosurgeon, Margarita or I couldn't predict was that a few minutes after my arrival, two urgent neuro-patients arrived in their big, colourful ambulances and were taken up to the neurosurgery department, where one of them was admitted . . . to *my* bed.

Margarita stood waiting nervously next to me on the A & E bed, which had been parked in the hallway, and I felt in limbo. After a few minutes a nurse came and took me into the huge, communal central room, where there was only a hand's distance between one bed and the next. A continuous coughing came from both sides and it felt like I was breathing in air from one ill person or another. There wasn't even room for Margarita to come and kiss me goodbye. I spent a few hours there and then, at five, when guests could walk in, I told Margarita to please talk to the nurses and put me back in the hallway, where I felt better.

~

The sounds of a different kind of emergency.

I had now spent three nights in the corridor of the A & E and I quickly discovered that there were plenty of other people who had opted to stay out here. The first person I made friends with was Eugenio, a big man of about my age, who proudly told me that, before checking in, he was drinking forty Ceres beers a day. Later I listened to the long-winded tales of a very tall transsexual, my eyes focused on the thick layers of make-up drizzling down her face. I don't know if she was actually talking to me or to the hallway in general. She seemed very unhappy with her treatment, but I noticed that when the old nuns passed by, she became very quiet, almost in reverence. I am sure that the Scientologists in LA would not like it, but here in Rome the nuns do still play a role – albeit an undefined one – in A & E.

The first night, there was an old man who felt he had to scream the story of his life as a Navy commander on a ship with trees, green trees . . . not red trees like the Italian flag . . . until 4 a.m., when some kind nurse decided to give him something to calm down that colour injustice and let us all sleep. I had several talks about addiction with my new friends and I gave my food to the transsexual, who I realized often came and hung out in A & E even if she didn't appear to like any part of the place.

When I told my neighbours about my illness, they all seemed sincerely surprised. Was I really weird for them or did I look too posh to be here? I could get away with my strange haircut in America, but here it might be too unusual. It was possible these were merely my anxieties, and here in A & E I was just another freak. I was completely bald on all sides of my head (thanks to the fashion police of radiotherapy), and while my hair pointed upward, my big beard flowed downward. None of my neighbours showed any interest in my illness, or maybe it was too intense for them, as every reference I made to death was ignored.

Yesterday, like most days, Bianca came and brought me food for lunch and it was one of those miraculous meals that only she can do. It was steamed fish and green beans, and after being inside for a whole day, it smelled even better. I guess I am a snob, but I can't bear eating the A & E food. I told my friends to keep an eye on my books and iPod, and while they were eating my dose of hospital food, I walked outside with Bianca and my mother and we sat down in the hot sun of Rome.

As I was telling them of my experiences, I noticed that Marianella had not sat down. She was stressed, and when she is like this, it means she has something burning in her stomach. She had left much of the management of my surgery to my doctor, Margarita, and she could no longer keep her emotions at bay.

Marianella shook her head slowly. 'Let's think about it. This is a hospital for hopeless cases. Is it really the right place for such a delicate operation, on your brain, while you are conscious? Those doctors told me that there will be eleven people in the operating room, and that some of them are still students.

'Martino, you have time to change your mind. We can go and talk with Professor Veronesi in Milan. For me, his European Institute of Oncology seems like a more reliable place than this. It is still a fluid situation and nobody can force you to stay. We can explore other possibilities.'

Keeping calm, and now with a piece of fish stuck in my throat, I told her, 'Mum, I am going ahead with this operation. I've made that decision and I'm not going to change my mind.' The discussion continued but I felt there was no way that I could convince her. Emotions were running high and as I said *No* for the tenth time, she walked away. I closed the box of food, handed it to my sister and did my best to meditate near the shadow of the building.

Today Eugenio left, and during the night I opened my eyes

and saw the transsexual also get up and walk out, with her skirt unfastened at the back and her long hair in a tangle. Who knows what will happen to them? While I am probably the one with the most dangerous illness clinically, I have the feeling that their mothers will be receiving a phone call about them much sooner than my mother will about me.*

~

Finally, now that I am in a regular ward with four 'similarly ill' people, I appreciate hugely the pillow on my bed, the water next to it, the closed door in the bathroom, and the stillness of the long hallway. Opposite me is a man who has already had a few operations on his back. He looked and spoke like a classic worker from the countryside outside Rome, but when his younger wife appeared at lunchtime, well dressed and with very sophisticated language, I realized I should not attempt to categorize people while I'm lying here.

We're all in pyjamas and we're all here because we have been living with our own individual dramas for a while. In here, each person creates their own hopes and demons to accompany them in this experience. I am no different from everyone around me, and though they all seem very private, I try to make small talk, at least with the two conscious people in the room. The old man lying at the end of the room does not make any sound, aside from the 'beep beep' of his machines, which are there to remind us that he is still alive, so I try not to think about him at all.

~

I have started the work to prepare for surgery, which should take place next Wednesday. There is also a series of scans and blood tests that will be used for some experimental protocols,

---

* Margarita: 'That summer, Rome was completely empty. Just me, your mother and Bianca. And you were in that strange hospital. My trips from our house to the hospital were always with the music of Amy Winehouse in the background. You had given me a CD with her songs. I remember that she died during that summer when you had your surgery. And I cried like crazy in that car to her music.'

which will be developed on the basis of the parts that will be extracted from my brain.

There is one experiment that I find particularly interesting, because the researchers are going to use parts of the cancer that currently lives in my head to create a dendritic vaccine. The way I understand it is that the cancerous pieces of my own brain will be transformed in a lab, and then get re-injected into my body, where they will be recognized as normal Aliens who just went out for a vacation. They will recognize and then attack the Alien cancerous cells from within, when they least expect it. I am excited about this, as it sounds like proper sci-fi stuff, and if it works, it will be the beginning of a new way of confronting cancer.

The discussion about doing the surgery while I am awake is still ongoing, but now that I have handed that call to the surgeon, my principal concern is to get some good pre-op meditation time and the permission to have a cameraman filming at least part of it. If I'm going to talk to people while parts of my brain are being cut off, I want to have a record of it. I'll use it for something. I don't know what yet, but come on! At some point, who knows, I'll see this as cool.

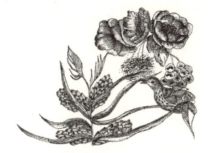

11

Brain Surgery While Awake

Rome, 2011

Today I have been walking through the different departments of the Policlinico hospital to undergo preparation for tomorrow's surgery. The pre-operation Functional Radiology Scan is done with a very high-tech machine surrounded by rows of rooms with very high-tech computers and screens with very high-tech images of different body parts. To make it even more high-tech, as part of the scan they have inserted an 'awake' part, where they monitor the movements of my brain while they ask me to give them a list of colours, animals, women's names and the names of cities. All this will result in a cool 3D scan, which will be used as a high-tech map for tomorrow's operation.

While I was walking through the endless series of doors, I noticed that there is a clock on the walls of every hallway in the hospital. Partly to avoid thinking of anything more intense, I pondered how these would illustrate the central function that time has in the organization of this medical institution, both symbolically and practically. The problem being when you notice, as I did on my walk, that the identical clocks indicate: 10.20 a.m. or p.m., 9.07 a.m. or p.m., 6.38 a.m. or p.m., 12.29 a.m. or p.m., and 4.04 a.m. or p.m. Not one single clock indicates the correct time.

In fact, upon further inspection, not one single clock is showing any sign of life. None of them has been plugged in or given a new battery. It is an odd sensation in this high-tech context of presumed precision to see time being treated with such indifference – it must be philosophically intentional. Otherwise what does it mean in a budget review for a hospital when the batteries for clocks are cut? What happens to our conception of space, time and the precision that we attribute to medical practice?

Further down the clock-less, time-less hallways, I met one of the surgeon's assistants, who was looking for me. He is a lovely-looking young man, who, when he becomes a surgeon himself, will be the ideal character that I was initially looking for. He is quite a bit younger than me and we talked informally with each other. He arrived with the instruments to give me a haircut and, as cutting only one part would look silly, I told him to take off everything that I still had on the top of my head. After he left, I looked at myself in the mirror and decided that I should cut the beard off, too. Go one hundred per cent clean into this adventure!

I just did that, and . . . it was a mistake. I really shouldn't have done it. All along the line, I have resisted the big dosages of my steroid medication, Bentelan. Even in A & E, when the nurses had been told to double my dosage, I had refused, but here the Prof has asked for it and so I am taking it. The result is that I have swelled up. I don't recognize my own face in the mirror and this hard-core haircut does not help.

Fortunately, a team of young women, assistant anaesthetists, arrived and took my thoughts away from that creature in the bathroom mirror. All three of them are quite short and wear matching brightly patterned, coloured headscarves. They, along with their teacher (I hope), will guide me through the process of waking me up and making me fall back asleep with full sedation during the operation. Their sidekick in this journey was my next guest: the neuropsychologist.

In this team her job is to make sure, in the twenty minutes when the anaesthetist gets me awake, that she asks me the right questions. Then the coloured-hat crew should push a magic-pill button and I'll be back asleep. When the surgeons are once more in a critical part of my head, they'll wake me up again so that the speech therapist can get me to rattle off another list of numbers backwards, months forward, and city names in any order.

I know that it is senseless to feel pressure before those questions. It's not a real exam. I went to university! I shouldn't be intimidated by a psychologist with a clipboard asking me the months of the year. Even if there is someone cutting bits off my brain. And even if I do get the answer wrong. That is not the point. In fact, that could be *the* point at that moment and they'll be able to draw their conclusions from the mistakes I make – cut more, less, differently? Is part of the problem that I find that speech therapist terribly pretty?

Nevertheless, my ego doesn't take a break, even on this occasion. Today, during the scan, I couldn't think of enough animal names and felt bad about it. I surprised myself by being unable to calculate 245 x 15 by long multiplication, and I was then surprised about being shocked about being surprised. But maybe having an overactive ego might be useful, as it could distract me from the fifteen people who will be in that room tomorrow, working with all their combined skills to cut the right parts out of my brain and leaving intact the ones that I'll still need to hopefully calculate 245 x 15 properly.

Off to sleep.

Tomorrow I'll start at 6 a.m. (my clock time) with some meditation, and then at 6.40 a.m. the anaesthetist will arrive for an 8 a.m. prompt start (Professor Santoro time).

~

As I finish my twenty-five-minute meditation, following the voice of the American hypnotherapist that I had saved in my computer, I see Margarita coming in. She looks tense. I am not. The other three men in my room are being woken up slowly by the nurses, who have come in to bring their morning pills. As my team arrives in the room, I say in a cheery voice, 'Hello, ladies and gentlemen, it's a beautiful day out here in Rome.' I kiss Margarita, who is still trying to make small talk, and then I am transferred on to a different bed and they start carrying me away. I watch the white squares on the ceiling pass slowly by, and after every three of them, a light interrupts them, until we stop at the second white square, after the fourth light.

Margarita's hand has been attached to mine throughout my whole journey on this travelling bed and as I raise my head to look at her, I see there is a metal barrier that has stopped our progress, so I guess I have arrived in the land of no return. Two big men lift me up and move me on to the other side of the barrier, while Margarita tries, for my sake, to keep her tears at bay with a brave smile.

Away I go. Pushed through a continuous series of metal doors, until I see the operation zone from afar. It looks quite cool. The three young women with their cheery headscarves are now fully covered by their green suits. I ask them if they're excited and they smile. They ask me if I mind, as they need to cut off some pieces from the legs and waist of my pyjamas. They look focused and move extremely quickly. One of them sticks a needle in my leg and another does the same, almost immediately, in my breast. I tell them that I am impressed, and that I hardly felt anything. God, I am talkative this morning. They show me a plastic box and explain to me that they will now make me fully unconscious. I assume that it will take a while to knock me out, but it takes only a few seconds.

My Spaceship has now taken off to explore the dangerous, uncharted area where eighty per cent of the Aliens still live. The journey is foggy, but fortunately I've got a map with me. I might not be able to see properly, but I will recognize those creatures when I get there. I am close, I can smell them. Just as I start bombing the hell out of the Aliens, I hear a radio sound coming through my ears. Wow, that's cool, I didn't know there was also a Wi-Fi radio in here. It is the voice of the American President, Barack Obama, who is giving me a pep talk.

'I know a lot of people are worried about the future. But here's what I also know: there will always be economic factors that we can't control – earthquakes, spikes in oil prices . . . But how we respond to those tests – that's entirely up to us . . .'

My battle in the Spaceship continues, and in fact it is being energized by this tale coming from the ears.

'We have had the determination to shape our future. And to move forward not only for this generation but for the next generation. We are going to need to summon that spirit today . . .'

Man, we are kicking ass, but . . . ouch. The Spaceship must have a malfunction, the computers are turning themselves on without following my mandate. Wow. My eyes open. I am completely awake. Awake in a way that . . . I have never been before. It's not that slow move into awareness. It's Bang! Reality.

My view is slightly obscured on the left-hand side by a blue sheet. I hear voices, over voices, over voices. I see that beautiful woman. The speech therapist. She is there with her white paper and a pen. I hear the voice of the surgeon, 'Hello, Martino.' He sounds quite cheery. In fact it sounds like everyone is having a good time. I tell them, 'It hurts,' and I hear brief laughter from someone out there.

The speech therapist gets closer and asks me, 'Martino, can you count from one to ten for me?' I obey, hoping that following her questions will distract me from the pain I feel in my head. Have they only turned on my brain? Because I don't seem to feel anything from my hands.

'Martino, now count backwards from ten.'

I get back into her groove. She is really pretty. Her legs seem to never end.

'Martino, can you tell me the alphabet . . . you know . . . A, B, C . . .' I follow her request until she says, 'Stop, thank you. Now can you do it backwards?'

I try . . . but quickly get lost on one of the letters. She moves on and asks me, with a strong Italian accent, 'Can you count to ten in English for me? Good, and now backwards?'

I say it very fast and then interject saying, 'It really, really hurts. Can you stop it? Please . . .' And just as quickly as I was awoken, my Spaceship starts up again.

I am kicking ass. I am tearing them apart. Those Aliens . . . Hhhhaaa . . . I am getting attacked from the other side, where we are starting to lose . . . something . . .

That was an emotional blow. Seeing good bits fall in the call of duty. I'll turn on the radio-phone to pep up the team. Come on, Obama . . . you are a pro.

'On Friday, we learned that the United States received a downgrade by one of the credit rating agencies . . . Our problems are imminently solvable . . . and we know what to do to solve them.'

If that is a pep talk, I am confused. I need an upper, not a . . . low . . . I am losing beats. I am losing speed. I don't know if the credit ratings were right. Maybe the President is lying, and maybe we are losing. I don't know. I am lost. If I stop, I'll die within a few months. That's what the statistics say.

Maybe I have to restart the machine. Maybe I'll substitute Obama with a quote from that good Italian philosopher, Antonio Gramsci, 'The crisis consists precisely in the fact that the old is dying and the new cannot be born.'

No shit! I am dying here! I need more than confidence and pep talks. I need some creative conflict negotiation. Maybe I have to find these Aliens some really nice houses in the brain of a fish who lives in the Mediterranean. Warm water, long summers. Access to North Africa. I'll put in a trip to Sharm el-Sheikh. There are gorgeous fish there. It's like a fish fashion show. I'll give you the same probabilities as those fish, who will be eaten by other sea creatures . . . which is 1 to 10,000 (as only one survives).

I am drained of all energy and afraid that I am losing. We should have negotiated something, invented a new solution. I never thought of my Aliens as creatures who are here as poor suckers, who also need a good place to procreate.

I have to park this Spaceship. If the war continues like this, everybody is going to die, both the Aliens and me. I'll tell them that I will change the music on my radio. I'll put on Glenn Gould piano riffs, as I'm sure they will cheer you up. No politics. No war! . . . Hurry up. Hit the brakes. Ouch . . .

~

I just woke up. I am in a hospital bed. It is night. I hear the tune of the computer next to me, measuring my heart rate. I am alive. I live. Why is it night? How long have I been here? I've got some material covering the left side of my face. Yep . . . now I know . . . I've got a big-ass, triple layer of fabric over my head. Good that I cut all my hair off. I am tired. I am alive. If I go to sleep, I will wake up again.

As I open my eyes, the first human person I see is my lovely nurse, who has come to put some more cortisone through my blood. I try to open my mouth and say good morning and nothing comes out. I try again . . . nothing. Have I lost my voice? I'll sleep some more and think about it later.

I open my eyes and my wife is there. My sister, too. I have thoughts that I can't manage to translate into sounds. I can still move my mouth, but it feels like it is under shock. That was intense. I didn't think I would remember it all so power-fully. My wife comes closer and tries to kiss the part of my face that is not covered. The movement of my bones somehow feels different. The weight is different.

I touch the fabric around my head, tap my finger on it and hear a foreign sound. It must be the fabric. What? Man! That's crazy (no pun intended), I don't remember my wife's name. She's a psychiatrist, she's my wife, she's the mother of my little boy. What's his name? Man!!! I don't have his name either? FUCK. What have they cut?*

That pretty logopedist only asked me for the numbers and the alphabet. She should have asked me for a list of people whose names I would also like to keep in my brain. 'I don't remember . . . I don't recall . . . I got no memory of anything at all.' That is a song that I like by . . .? He was big in the 1980s. He is still cool. He did this tour while wearing a suit that was twice as big as him, and so his head seemed really small over his body. He did a whole show dressed like that. What's happening in my head? What has been cut away? Have I won? Or have I lost?

Fortunately, that question was promptly resolved with the arrival of the brain surgeon, who walked into the room followed by a posse of young men, and that sweet girl. The one who told me that she was trying to enter into the world of neuro-surgeons but was finding it almost impossible, as it is a men's

---

* Margarita: 'When you woke up from that operation and they asked you the name of your wife, and you could not remember, it really hurt me. How is it possible that he does not remember? I was there and I thought, who is this person? Who are we? Then I realized that it was a wider problem but . . . it was the end.'

club. Was she there last night? I would very much like to hear the woman's point of view of how the operation has gone. How I did in my scene. That is . . . if I could talk.

The Prof walked past me with his crew and went to see the older man in the back of the room. Then he passed by the man opposite me, who was recovering from an operation on his back. Then he stopped in front of me. He smiled and asked me how I was doing. I moved my mouth to speak and nothing came out. I didn't remember the words. Or maybe I just . . . I don't know. He smiled, touched my hand and with a confident smile walked away. His body language was saying, 'All is good. You look good. We did a good job and I'm proud of it.'

I try to talk but almost nothing comes out. 'I . . .' 'Po . . .' . . . It doesn't work. I need a nap.

~

I have regained some of my speech. I can make a sentence, but don't remember . . . anything. My wife tells me her name, 'Margarita'. It's obvious, yes. She asks me for the name of the street where we live and I try for a few seconds. I am sure that I had it saved in at least twenty parts of my brain. I have to get it.

'Via Braccio da Montone,' she says. She continues like that until, frustrated, I tell her to stop.

~

The young and handsome surgeon-to-be, and the young woman who had her hopes on being one, came by to check on me and change the material that I have on my head. It was nice to take it off. I touched my head and the response to the contact felt different. As if I had a new piece attached. I told them that I had tried to read something and my eyes went crazy and I couldn't see more than two letters at a time. They seemed curious, but explained that after such an operation, many things are provoked and affected.

'Will I get it back?'

They looked at each other and the voice of the young lad became more serious, as he said, 'If you had been a builder, someone who works with his body and not with his brain every day, then I would say, no, you will not get it back. But as your work is to read, it could be that . . . with time . . . it can get at least a bit better. I haven't encountered this about reading, but in other situations, that's how it works.'

My mother arrived for lunch with my sister. They brought me some decent food and my mother gave me a magazine for children who are just starting to read. I tried a few of the exercises, but quickly knew that it wasn't for me. I don't have the memory to know which letter was at the beginning of the word. It took me twenty seconds to read 'Dog', and so I guess I will have to meditate . . . a lot.

~

Writing, right after having come out of a twenty-five-minute meditation, looks like this. My fingers do their instinctive touch-type, which is already pretty cool. I close my eyes and the thoughts translate into words. They concern themselves with what is happening in the present, now. The wife of that man in front of me. She is helping him put on his white T-shirt, and her smile tells me that she is conscious that she has not done this for years, since their children were small.

My mind only wanders through the present and the day ahead. What I don't do is mix up different ideas and thoughts and start bouncing between them. It is like having pressed 'force quit' on everything in my computer and noticing that now the software operates better as I open my necessary apps. My recent and ancient history are still there but, at least for a while, I can embrace thoughts on a new, clean piece of paper.

I don't bother with the text that is coming out, as I can't read it right now. At some point, I'll come back and hopefully be able to read this, and I'll remember the weird sensation that I'm having. This text and I, we're starting a different relationship. That is pretty bloody obvious. I like the fact that a British word just popped out of my fingers as a response to those emotions. 'Bloody hell', rather than 'What the fuck' – somehow it's gentler.

I just said goodbye to that man who occupied the bed opposite. He and his lovely wife were laughing as they walked away, with her attempting to prop up his, much taller, shoulder. I do hope that the person who is going to take his place will be conscious. That man by the window . . . he makes me think that I have to meditate some more. I can't believe that I'll actually be out in a day. Walking the streets of Rome with this big wrapped-up white sheet on my head.

~

What do you think about that? Writing without reading after a meditation feels like producing gobbledygook, but also all right. I guess I used to do it when I woke up from dreams when I was younger, or rather, healthier. It only took a few minutes of listening to the yells coming from some patient in the corridor for me to notice that the app, where all the anxieties are stored, had opened itself up. I am sure I can get this computer to read me what I am writing. I simply have to find the right button, but as there seems to be only text on the screen in front of me . . . I will never find it. Yes. I'll meditate again, a lot.

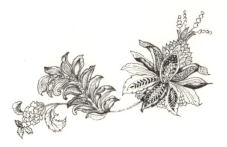

12

A Home, a Child and Work

Rome, London and Miro, 2006–10

It was a hot summer in Rome, and as I finished putting together my experimental Thai salad infusion, I went up to the first floor of our cute little house with my hands still wet, and looked at Margarita sitting at the table by the window. She looked like she was having such an intense relationship with those three textbooks in front of her that I put my hand on her shoulder and asked her very quietly, 'How's it going? How much more do you have to do?'

173

She smiled back at me and said, 'Well, I still have to review Blood and Lymph, Musculoskeletal Infections, Skin, Homeostatic Endocrine, Neurological, Respiratory, Renal, Urological, Genito-urinary and Cardiovascular . . .'

This equivalency exam, which she had to pass to get her medical accreditation in Italy, sounded ridiculous to me, as there were too many words that meant absolutely nothing to me. I was hugely impressed by her ability to hold so much foreign information in her head, and I knew that I would never dare put myself in that situation. With a laugh, I said, 'And then you are done?'

She stood up and sighed. 'Then I also have to do the Digestive and Reproductive system. The only one that I'm absolutely sure about is Psychiatry and Mental Health, but I bet you that I'll end up failing the exam for exactly a question about that. They'll ask me about a tiny little detail that almost never occurs or a strange developmental problem that I can't remember.'

'Is becoming a doctor all theory?'

'Well, while I was at school I had to do a residency in every one of those subjects . . .'

'Even brain surgery?'

'Yes, I didn't like it at all as we had to spend a whole day with a dead body, and it smelled awful.'

I held her arm as we walked downstairs to lunch. 'You really don't seem happy, my love.'

Almost in tears, she replied, 'I really don't want to do this again . . .'

Ever since we'd met, I'd tried to support her by negotiating with the chaotic and cruel bureaucracy of Italy, particularly towards non-European émigrés, but sadly I couldn't do much to help with this academic issue of medicine. And I knew that, in fact, she had never wanted to do medicine at all.

Margarita's mother had explained many times to her that, as an architect, making drawings was only a small part of her profession, and she was sure that her daughter wouldn't be happy spending most of her time with construction workers, or making budgets.

I guess that it was exactly the opposite of how my sister and I were raised. I'll always remember when I was living in Brixton, shortly after I'd finished my MPhil at Cambridge, my mother called me and with no irony at all told me, 'I'm proud of you, since it seems that in bartending you've found a profession that makes you happy.' That call still resonates in my head and makes me think that as children we all have fun creating things, but as we grow up, most of us start fearing the judgement of the group and the family.

The designs that Margarita had drawn on paper and pasted down our stairs, expressed clearly to me that she was only truly at peace when she was creating art, and that at thirty-three years old she had still not given up on her dream. What her parents had not seen was her sitting outside on our little street, blissfully happy, engrossed in the interior design magazines that I would bring back to her from London. The work and energy that she was putting into conceptualizing our new apartment made it clear to me that her real love lay in the world that existed in those magazines.

~

After Margarita passed her Italian medicine equivalency exam, we decided to move into our still only semi-reconstructed apartment. While for me – a big, burly man – all the first-generation African and North African immigrants who lived in our new neighbourhood were simply a new addition to the Rome that I had grown up with, I appreciated that it took quite a bit of effort for Margarita to make peace with the 'rough sides' of our new life.

In the evenings and weekends, I tried to keep her attention on the artful bespoke designs that we could create together for all the rooms, and even on our gigantic terrace, which in Rome one can use at least nine months of the year. I believed that it was a perfect project for us in every way, as it made us focus on our future together.

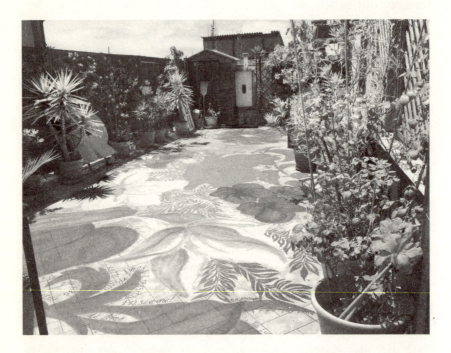

How to resolve all the problems in our house with so little money was an exciting game for us, and all our efforts and emotions went into this venture. We found some metal builders who, for a third of the price that we had been quoted by the big companies, built us a set of stairs that allowed us to go comfortably from the apartment to the terrace. Another group, after initially shaking their heads that it would be impossible, enjoyed creating an intentionally crooked bookcase for us, and as we had only the terrace over our head, we put up a fire-burning (*Alex . . . help me . . .*) place (where you put wood, make fire and cook).

Rather than creating a 2 Many Executives hub in Italy, I had decided to join forces with Matteo's company, Roma Film. He knew the Italian film world much better than I did, and was an expert at putting in applications for the various European funds.

One of the projects that I had developed in Bologna which was still dear to me was called *Valvorama*. It was an animated feature film set in the world of Italian comic books, which for the first time ever would make various characters from different historical periods interact with each other.

The main character of the story was the 1980s Italian classic Massimo Zanardi, created by Andrea Pazienza, and the brief synopsis for the film was: 'After having crossed paths and made chaos in the various worlds of other famous historical comic book characters, in his desperate attempts to become independent from his own author, Zanardi realizes that there are rules everywhere that he does not want to accept, and he has to come back to embrace his author, finally understanding that the creativity and uniqueness of his creator was the thing that had given him freedom.'

This was how we presented the story to the various European funding bodies, but the ending of our film was going to be a bit different. In our version of the story, as Zanardi comes back to his world, he realizes that his author, Pazienza, is dead due to a heroin overdose and he has to accept his place in a wonderful library, filled with various historical comic-book characters.

Our Bologna-based director, Francesco Merini, accepted that I was busy renovating my apartment and often came down to Rome to work on the story with me, while Margarita was painting the walls of our bathroom, inspired by the radical style of American artist Robert Rauschenberg. I sat with Francesco in the (still white) living room, organizing the plot around the famous historical characters that, after quite a bit of wheedling and charming, we had obtained permission to use in our film.

Matteo, Francesco and I spent a few days in the countryside, talking and hanging out with the girlfriend of Pazienza, who had the rights for our main character. While listening to her, I realized that a good part of my interest in developing this film, perhaps unconsciously, was the strong similarity between the character of Zanardi and his author, and Russell. I suspect that writing has always been an unconscious path of self-therapy for me. In this particular case, it was the tale of an unruly, mad, charming creature that found love through rebellion and later died from an overdose of heroin.

In the evening, I would rush back home to continue building our dream house and while Margarita was painting designs around the windows, inspired by the photographs we'd taken during a romantic weekend in Naples, I hung up various cabinets on the walls in the kitchen. I mixed pieces from the low-budget Swedish design supermarket with some fixtures that the local workers had helped me to make, and in this way we managed to put together a really striking and unusual kitchen.

Describing all the architectural details of our house is important, because later on in this story *(and I have to make a note of this, otherwise I am sure I will forget about it)*, somewhere towards the end of this book, what will happen is that this very beautiful and artful kitchen is going to fall down. Almost like a perfect film set, it will collapse on to Margarita, fortunately without causing her any actual physical damage. Yes, all our dreams and our artistic expressions of love for each other, every detail of that apartment, its terrace and the relationships with the people in the neighbourhood, will be handed over to new tenants, in exchange for money.

This is a note that I should remember to erase, as it is too sad, at least here, for this part of the story.

During the reconstruction of our house, I had made sure that there were wires throughout the whole apartment that would allow me to turn music on in every room, including the terrace and the bathroom, and also another one that hooked up to a projector on the ceiling of the living room, from which we could watch proper films in the evening when it got dark. I remember very clearly one evening, lying on the couch with all the house lights turned off and both of us with a glass of red wine, choosing a film from my stash of DVDs by an American director, Julian Schnabel, whose work we both loved.

It was called *The Diving Bell and the Butterfly*, and his previous film about a homosexual writer in Cuba had been in English, so I turned it on without worrying about the subtitles, but as the film started, I realized that it was in French and the only subtitles on the scratched copy that I had picked up at the market in Skopje were in Serbo-Croatian.

Margarita started reading the Serbo-Croatian and simultaneously translating it to me in Italian, allowing me to follow this true story of a man who, from his normal, successful life, falls into an illness that takes away the control of his whole body. Holding our heads close to each other, and hearing the soft sound of her voice in my ear, made this already dramatic romance even more poignant for me.

As the main character discovers that the only part of his body he can still control is one of his eyes, he finds a system, together with an assistant at the hospital, that allows him to fully communicate with the people around him. He and his family have to slowly come to terms with his illness and, somehow, even find moments in which they have peace. The camerawork on this film is outstanding, as it never lets you feel his handicap, and in fact he often narrates the world as he experiences it from his point of view, with his old voice. I have re-watched this film recently alone, without the voice of Margarita speaking into my ear, and while it is still stunning, I now find it a much sadder tale.

In Rome, our main means of transport was Margarita's car, a little Peugeot Punto (*thanks, Alex*) with Macedonian plates, and there was a period when every week I would drive Margarita, with a big, pregnant belly, up and down the hills outside Rome, where she supervised ten patients who were living together in a mental home, with the assistance of two nurses. Although her salary was unreliable, she had at least started to put a foot down in the world of Italian psychiatry and she had to accept all the jobs that the older colleagues did not want to do.

While she was meeting her patients, one by one in her office, I would sit outdoors to smoke a cigarette with some of them, who were glad to have someone from the outside they could talk to. I had never spent so much time with people who really were living in a parallel universe and I became intrigued by each one of them and their relationships with one another. I tried to understand that for Margarita, aside from the economic and professional difficulties here in Rome, the idea of living all her life with mentally ill patients was depressing, but every moment that I was there with those people made me appreciate her even more.

The schedule of my 2 Many Executives and Roma Film trips was often put together around the various film festivals, where we would find many other producers and financiers. The more important ones for us were the Berlin, Venice and Cannes film festivals, as we were trying to produce films together with other European countries.

While Margarita came with me a few times to the festivals and loved the atmosphere, George Lenz found the walk through the Cannes film market a horrible experience, as his artistic sensibilities were confronted with rows of companies from all over the world, sitting next to a bunch of film posters, like butchers in front of their meat. The smell was a bit less intense, but the reality almost identical to any other kind of market. 'A bunch of this and a bunch of that, perhaps, and if you want to buy my big film, then you will also have to take these little ones, which you can use and distribute as you please.'

Even if our child was conceived in that city, we never thought of giving him a French name. Although we ran through all the Italian and Macedonian names for our baby, we could not find one that inspired us and we decided to wait for him to be born, so we could ask him what he would like. The hospital that we had chosen was the most beautiful and romantic building that anyone could dream of. It is on the Isola Tiberina, which is a tiny island in the middle of the River Tiber.

After he was born, I was the first person to clean him and get him dressed. Initially I had no idea how to pick up or touch a child, but as soon as I saw him I felt secure. I wandered through that hospital with my little boy lying face down on my right arm, moving up and down like an aeroplane, floating curiously through his new world.

He was a calm child from the very beginning, expressing his needs with a minimum of screams or tears. One morning I looked out from the window of Margarita's hospital room, and as the tops of the churches were grabbing the first glimpse of the day, I prayed that this miraculous little creature would be blessed with love, joy and good health. Margarita turned her head in my direction and, almost overcome by the moment, she pointed towards our little boy's eyes, which were focused on her face with a pure expression of love.

We had told our parents that we wanted to live without them for the first few days of this boy's life. So, apart from our friends, whom we had invited, the only people that broke the rules and came were my Uncle Antonio and his friend Anna Carli. I had not thought about it, but this little creature had a particular importance for Antonio's vision of the Sclavi family, as he was the first born. Although he had been the director of Unicef in Italy, he was afraid of touching little children; rather than picking him up, he started talking to us for the first time about his grandparents and the concept of legacy and family, which I found simultaneously a strange and a sweet thing to do.

Before leaving the hospital, we had to give our little boy a name, but now that we had lived with him for two days, it was not a problem at all. We looked at each other and knew that he was our little boy Miro. We had never heard of the name, apart from the Spanish artist Joan Miró, or the abbreviation of names like Miroslav or Vladimiro. We walked out of the hospital on a sunny winter's day, crossed the river to the Jewish Ghetto and brought Miro to our home.

Thanks to Miro's tranquil temperament and Margarita's joy,

the first years of his life were beautifully calm. We took him with us to art galleries and parties and he looked curiously at the world and then without too much effort went to sleep. We talked to a few friends with children and it did seem that, beyond our obvious love for our son, we had an extraordinarily peaceful child.

Sadly, it was 2009 and the global financial crisis was overwhelming the economy. The Italian projects that I had spent so much effort in developing were losing any semblance of hope. The ideas were too ambitious for this period of uncertainty, where the only movies to be financed would be the ones from the established producers, and the ones from the super-established, mainstream producers. Did I just say that twice? Yes, because it became so obvious that Matteo, during a trip to France, decided to drop the whole idea of making films and started working with an old English-Italian friend making furniture. The only hopes for 2 Many Executives lay in London, so we set up a proper office in the centre of town with a few bedrooms where, if we wanted the company to function, I would have to invest most of my time.

I brought Miro and Margarita with me to London a few times and tried to show my wife the positive sides of my new existence in England. Moving from Skopje (less than one million residents) to Rome (a bit over three million) had already been a big jump for Margarita, so in proposing the option of London (something over twelve million), I was aware that it could be too much for her.

If she were to move here with a man like me, who did not have a classic steady job, she would have to start once again with a new (even if slightly less overwhelming) set of exams for her medical degree. That was already a huge barrier. Perhaps if I had a highly remunerated 'fixed' job that would allow her to focus on her interior design, then I could possibly negotiate with her, but that was not on the cards at the moment.

In our lovely Roman neighbourhood of Pigneto, gentrification was in full swing, and though the wider Italian economy appeared to be collapsing, there were new bars being opened on every street. While I spent my time in London, Margarita had started to become friends with a group of people in the neighbourhood who shared her love for art, design and fashion. Whenever I returned to Rome with toys for Miro and some new designer clothes for Margarita, it became more difficult for us to connect emotionally. For me the priority was to spend quality time with her and with Miro, and though her new friends did seem nice, I was not really interested in spending our rare evenings out listening to other voices. The lonesomeness of my life, living alone in my office in London, was something that I had created and that I could not really share with my wife, as I was the one that had to fix it. Fair enough, I guess.

Knowing that many people in her new group of friends – and sometimes it seemed everyone in their forties – were going through divorces, we were aware of the risk that we were running by increasing the distance between us. While I was in Rome, I often tried talking with my friends about finding a new job there, but they were astonished by this idea. Everyone who could was getting out of town, and the ones that stayed were keeping their hands tightly on whatever job they had, so I just had to make my wife appreciate the flexibility that I had, being the boss of my own international company.

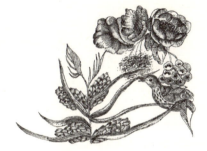

13

Being a Patient as a Job

Rome, August 2011

While I was lying in that hospital bed, I had nurses checking me continuously to monitor that my doses were dropping into my veins at exactly the right rhythm, and if I felt that my pain was rising, they would bring me the pills to make it all go away. I was safe, I was being taken care of. If I could not get a word out of my mouth they would wait, put their hand on mine and by moving their head as a sign of calm and patience, allow me to stop, breathe and start again with my search for a missing piece of language.

185

Now that I'm back in the real world, outside the Policlinico hospital, I realize that I didn't appreciate the nurses enough in my time there. Even though it's a hot summer, I always try to wear a hat in order not to scare the world around me, and for most people going about their daily routine, I am just a big fat dude with a hat. No one comes to check up on me and there's no reason to do so. I guess I am, for them, a 'normal person'. While in reality I am my old self, but stuck in the body of a big bear, with the intellect of a sheep.

Where did my memory go? Is it called memory? Is that the right word? What is it? Names of fruits, or . . . or vegetables . . . what are the vegetables that I actually remember? Tomatoes, potatoes . . . those are cool, but I don't seem to associate words and . . . physical matter. Since Miro is in nursery, I ask Margarita to give me a list of things that I should buy from the market. I try to read her words and even though they are not in Serbo-Croatian, which she occasionally uses for her own notes, I can't make any sense of them.

I want to do it. I want to go and buy fruit and vegetables. I want to regain control of my existence, of my body, of my mind, and so I put her little piece of paper in my pocket, close the door behind me and walk down the stairs.

I stride down the street and across a pathway that brings me over the train tracks and into the central part of our neighbourhood, Pigneto. There in the pedestrian area, six days a week, I can find a row of fruit and vegetable stands. By now I know the ones that I like. I'm sure I didn't originally choose them for the quality of their produce, because they're all very similar and my knowledge of fruit and vegetables is not sophisticated enough to be able to make a proper assessment. In fact, as I walk through the crowd, I realize that I've selected these stands because their owners have a good sense of humour, and when I'm there waiting for my turn, they entertain me with their repertoire.

Many of the stands are run by husband-and-wife teams, who

all seem like perfectly matched couples. While the women are cutting and preparing the vegetables, the men serve, and often break into their sales pitch: 'Apppples! They're good for you! They make you feel fantastic. Appples! Six apples for one Euro. Come and try them!'

The man working on the stand next door ignores the apple song and cockily chimes in with, 'Oranges . . . Oranges for you . . .' He looks at me, and continues loudly, 'You can juice them, or you can eat them as they are. Here . . .' He pulls out a knife and cuts one in half to show me the red flesh inside. How can I not buy them? I need to be good to my body and this is definitely good for me.

I notice that he hasn't recognized me. Is it because he's performing? More probably, it's because the cortisone that I inject every morning and night has transformed my face, belly and legs into a completely different human being. Now that I think about it, I'm pleased that I don't get recognized. I would much rather that people remember me as the handsome, charming man that used to come a few times a week and engage in their word games.

In fact, in July, I was here with a funny haircut and a big beard, and that guy had recognized me and we did have a chat. Now, thanks to cortisone, I feel like the Elephant Man. I ignore Margarita's list and point my finger to the different types of vegetables laid out on his stand. He follows me with his own hand, just asking me for quantities and not for names, picks up all the fruits and bags them up for me, then he turns his head to the side, making his wife aware of my presence.

As she ties some bundles of greens together, she turns to look at me, stares for a second, and then tries to clean her hands by rubbing them on her trousers, while walking towards me. She looks shocked, and doesn't know whether to hug me with her dirty hands. In the end she raises her hands in the air as a sign of welcome.

'I can't hug you, but . . . I would . . . I would,' she says and with a huge smile, slightly tinged with fear, asks me how I am doing. What can I say to a person like that? Someone I have known for a long time, but with whom I have never spoken about anything apart from the weather or . . . the weather.

I give her a brief synopsis of my adventure and raise my shoulders in a gesture of 'What can you do?' She grabs a fruit, gives it to me with a smile and says, 'I'm glad you're well again. All of us here in the market have been praying for you.'

I didn't know, but the news of my illness has done the rounds in my hood. People don't trust themselves to approach me, but now that I know, I can read the movement of their eyes, which follow me as I walk, and I see them move their heads up and down, as an unspoken sign of 'glad that you're alive'.

I am told that the Prof, a local character, whom I have only ever seen sitting alone, drinking his glass of white wine in the various bars of the neighbourhood, has been the one who has been most worried about me, and has been continuously asking my friends for news.

As I pass by the wine shop and see him sitting outside, I put down my bags and ask him if I can sit on the bench next to him. He smiles awkwardly at me and says, 'Can I buy you a glass? . . . White?'

I smile back at him. 'Don't worry, I just drink water.'

Without hesitation he stands up and comes back with a plastic glass filled with sparkling water. Up until now our communication had been limited to looking at each other and raising our hands while crossing paths, but now I feel at ease sitting next to him. His beard is neatly trimmed and he always wears a suit, with a tie – even in summer – which I think is part of the reason why everyone calls him the Prof.

Not sure if he is actually a professor and of what, I tell him a bit of my chaotic experience in A & E at the Policlinico hospital, and of the fantastic nurses I met there, who had endless patience for all kinds of people. He keeps on smiling sincerely and when he does speak he is very quiet and keeps his eyes focused on his plastic cup. While we are both looking at the cars passing by in front of us, I force myself to stay quiet and embrace the awkwardness of that minute with joy.

Following his slow rhythm, I recognize a stark similarity to meditation. Is he the neighbourhood's version of a Tibetan Buddhist monk? Or is he just a mental case who has been embraced by the family unit of our streets? Our realities may be a million miles away from each other, but at that moment, nothing is complex or problematic.

As I finish off my glass and stand up, I notice that his hand is touching my arm. Instinctively I find myself turning my body around and making contact with him. Our arms are clasped and it ends up feeling as if we're soldiers saying goodbye before going back home. Walking down the road, I turn around and while attempting to raise my hand in a Che Guevara-type, clenched-hand salute, I see that I am waving about a bag of vegetables, which makes us both smile at my silliness.

It was great to sit there and feel the very human side of my neighbourhood, the substrata of the bigger city. It is these details of the human condition, these social minutiae, that make me feel that I am at home. There might be many problems here, and it can't be compared to my dreamy reality of Los Angeles, but it is home, a concept that I don't think I've ever treasured as much as I do now.

~

Just a few months after the operation on my brain, I notice that it's harder for me to find my various doctors at the hospital. I presume they're no longer so interested in my progress. They have an endless number of patients and, so long as I'm fine, why should they occupy their precious time with me, a non-ill person? The only thing I can do, every twenty-eight days, is visit the team of neurosurgeons who cut my brain into bits, and while they're giving me a new stash of pills, I ask them some questions.

My team, composed of Margarita, my mother and myself,

have been walking about knocking on various doors, trying to find some clarity from someone. I know that Margarita, rather than talking loudly, particularly in social events, listens attentively to people, a skill that fits her psychiatrist persona perfectly. It also makes her engage magically with doctors on a different level. In fact, tomorrow we're going to meet the chief of the oncology department of the Policlinico hospital, whose private phone number Margarita has obtained from a couple of Italian doctors whom she met during an art exhibition in LA. Knowing how to socialize with other doctors at such events does make a huge difference. Margarita reassures me that, even in the more chaotic reality of Italy, I will continue to be in touch with the best staff and for that, once again, I have to thank the socialite who is my wife.

There is continuous anxiety in my camp because, while Margarita remains steadfast and follows the advice of her old and experienced teacher, Ada Francia, my mother cannot find peace. Ada, who has always tried to stay out of our decisions, obviously trusts the opinion of her friend, the neurosurgeon who operated on me. At the moment, I'm being followed up by his team, who believe the operation was successful in removing the cancer, and that soon they will be able to take me off the expensive cancer drug Temodal and leave me with the anti-epileptic one that is standard after such an excision.

I would love to remember the names of all the people who have been taking care of my brain, but at least for now, their ego has to accept that they're parked right next to all the other lovely bits and pieces that they happened to take away from my head.

So what am I to do, when the super-head of oncology at the hospital, Professor Cortesi, whose private number we were given by those friends in LA, looks me straight in the eye and tells me that, if I stop taking the Temodal, I will be travelling alone in the world of statistics for this illness? I like him, but I do understand what he's telling me: there is absolutely no reason, according to him, why my life will not come to an end in six to nine months from now.

What can I do with that information? I am surrounded by too many options, and for me two are already too many. How do I make a choice about something like this? For the moment, I've found a trick that allows me to not make that decision and I'm happy with that. As long as the surgeon's team is still giving me the same high dosages of Temodal, I am fine.

Yesterday I tried to sneak into Cortesi's office, which is always packed with older ladies complaining about their pain while waiting for their turn, and I asked him, on the go, if he could please look quickly at my bi-weekly blood results and give me his opinion. I realize now that I can't do that. I put him on the spot, and as his world is oncology, most other people there are probably in situations that are just as urgent as mine. How can I chill out, though? When are *they* all predicted to die? Before or after me?

Here in the radiology department, under the building where I was operated on, I wait. I am sitting here, surrounded by a bunch of people who all think that their illness is more hard-core than anyone else's. We're all waiting for the assistant to the surgeon, who will give us our doses. Now that I think about it, why does Oncology have all the old women, while the radio-surgeons' patients are almost all men? Where would I rather be? Those women sitting in Professor Cortesi's department seem unfriendly. On the other hand, I have always preferred hanging out with women.

Maybe it's because I've always been bad at playing football. Or simply that I like the company of women more than men. I did have a brief moment in college when I thought I should at least give my gay side a try, but my physical reaction was so strong that I never tried it again. Now we're all waiting here, sitting next to each other for hours at a time, and none of us even has a chat about football. The assistant usually pops down about forty minutes after we've arrived, at times even later than that. He always gives us all the same time for our meeting, which keeps us continuously checking who will be going next, and who has arrived first.

There's a guy doing the paperwork at the entrance, who always seems to have the correct information about when we should expect our doctor to turn up. He has misshapen legs, but I've noticed there are a surprisingly large number of disabled people working in Italian public hospitals. While in one of those big American hospitals these people would be marginalized, here they are the managers and the assistants. They have a certain grade of power that gives them respect.

Am I disabled too? A man who can't read, can't remember any important words, names or numbers. Sometimes I have a date in mind – let's say the 13th – but then, when I tell someone about it to make a date, out of my mouth comes 'forty-three', and sadly, until someone points it out, I'm not aware of it. I'm not sure what I've just said. What was that number again? I've even forgotten it while I'm trying to make this point, to explain it, and I'm really concentrating. Let's see . . . yes, it was 1 . . . 3 . . . 13th.

When I come to the hospital and try to manage in this world, I simply tell Miro, 'Daddy's going to work.' What else can I tell him? I'm spending most of my time here, with the ill people, and I'm slowly getting used to being part of their team. Am I proud of that? Well, not at the moment, but I hope that writing this book might help me make peace with my new identity.

My impatience brings me to self-manage my relationship with my pills. I know it's not advisable and probably not an intelligent way of living with this new reality, but I can't help it. Often, what the doctors tell me doesn't sound sincere. It's part of their protocol and I can't feel there's anything standard in my illness. Since my operation in LA, I've been taking an anti-epileptic pill every morning. I've been told by several people that after an operation like mine, the probabilities of getting an epileptic attack are high, but recently I forgot to take those pills for a few days, and nothing happened. I now consciously forget them, and still nothing happens. Am I just waiting for the epileptic attack to happen, to feel a reaction? I don't know, but considering my relationship with numbers and probabilities these days, I've decided to stop taking them, and that's it.

In the same way, I recently decided to take the cortisone out of my life, and since I did that, my body has gone crazy. All these medicines continue to change every week, depending on what the doctor thinks and how badly my body is reacting to them. No one is particularly surprised that my emotions are shooting up and down as well. I don't want to eat and I want to sleep every day. Is this due to my lack of cortisone?

I did a round of checks with different doctors and have been told that my constant tiredness is probably due to the fact that my thyroid is damaged. I looked into this and the thyroid is a small, butterfly-shaped gland in my neck. It's quite important, because it produces several key hormones that help oxygen to enter cells and are the centrepiece of the body's metabolism.

The oncologists say that it has nothing to do with the pills, the operation or anything else, which I cannot believe. How come my whole body has started going crazy on me at exactly the same time? These things are not random. In any case, I'm now on 100 milligrams a day of Eutirox (the thyroid substitute) and my blood results are better. I still have headaches and am tired, though.

~

When I take Miro to the park, he immediately runs towards the swings, I push him up and down, and he never gets bored with it. I've been trying to explain to him the way the swing works, and how, by moving his body forward with his legs and then backwards, he will have more fun and be independent from me. Standing and pushing is not my favourite activity at the moment, so yesterday I tried to interest him in another game. Since he is still light, I picked him up and put him on the slide.

When he looked at me, all excited, as he ran up the stairs to glide back down, I asked myself if I was being lazy and using the powerful drugs that make me feel exhausted as an excuse. Every single time that Miro landed and stood up from that grey metal slide, he paused for a split second, our eyes met, and we both smiled with the same ridiculous joy. 'Yes, do more!' The thought of having a Miro who might have to live without his father is . . . difficult. Much more so than thoughts of my own death.

In the past six months, I've been neglecting my relationship with him. I've been napping a lot – both from physical need and as a psychological escape. There is more competition to get Miro time, as playing and particularly snuggling in bed with him in the evening is much needed by everyone. I understand that both his grandmothers and Margarita need to find refuge from my continuous stress. I would love to read him a book, or at least be able to stay in his fantastic world for longer amounts of time. I want to be independent, to see my family do their own thing, without thinking of me. I want to have my body back!

He's really the only person who doesn't care that I am tired or ill. I think he is aware, but has no issue with it. He expresses very clearly what he wants and needs, but when he realizes that Dad can't help him, he doesn't make me feel guilty about it. But I do feel guilty. I want to use every single moment that I have with him; I want to resolve all his problems and discover all his desires. When I need to nap, I give him paper, colours and a promise that when he has finished and Daddy has woken up – in twenty minutes – we can go out on our next adventure.

~

Something kind of bad has happened. I went, as usual, to meet the neurology assistant to pick up my pills. He knows that I've been talking to Cortesi and simply ignores it, which is a blessing.

As long as you don't openly discuss the problem, it can be ignored. But doctors do become upset when you start doubting their choices, or their work, and that's fair enough. This time I was the one to make a mistake.

It was one of those days when I had to go downstairs, to the basement of the building where I had been operated on, to pick up my dose of Temodal, and because I knew that I was going to wait for a long while down there, I brought my mother along, who had just arrived in Rome a few days before, from . . . wherever she had been giving her lectures on how to resolve conflicts.

We chatted for a while and then I closed my eyes and had a quick nap, while she kept an eye on the assistant's door down the hall. When we finally got in, I was still half asleep and something happened. I'm not sure how, but my mother was criticizing the assistant for something and he was really short-tempered with her, which caused her to tell him, 'We're actually following what Cortesi is saying, so the two of you should talk to each other!'

He tried to keep his cool, but did not manage it very well. He gave me my dose of Temodal, then said, 'Next time you go to Oncology to pick up your pills,' and showed us out, without the usual paperwork that I need to get my blood tests done for the next meeting.

This situation really stressed me out. The next day, I walked through Cortesi's offices, wanting to have an unbooked appointment in order to tell him what had happened. He seemed enraged, and I think it wasn't only about my arrogant arrival (though that was a good part of it), because it felt as if something has been brewing between the two departments that my mother and I have unconsciously managed to bring out into the open.

For some time now, I've been having a rather complex and stressful relationship with my wife. Here in Rome, Margarita is continuously carrying with her all the stress of my illness and she doesn't have many people with whom she can talk about it. She's the only person who has managed to negotiate with all the different political spheres of my hospital, and this latest turn of events (I am now officially in the hands of Dr Cortesi and the oncology department) has somehow tipped her over the brink. She is not a happy person in any way, and I feel that nothing I am trying is helping her.

For months now my wife and I have been moving about the three rooms of our house without ever really recognizing the other human who occasionally crosses our path while in search of a snack in the fridge. And while I see her grabbing and cracking a piece of chocolate I open up the tin of anchovies.

While writing about these events I can talk about my Aliens, cancer and even the concept of my imminent death with a certain sense of humour, but I have realized that when these thoughts come out of my mouth, they just create emotional and physical walls. Yes, I know, they are not romantic words and I have tried, but I really can't censor myself all the time in my own home.

When I encounter my new body in the mirror I am reminded that it has a good potential for repulsion, but I can't do much about the fact that it still continues to have human urges. Can that really be the ultimate cause of our marital problems? Can it? You remember that I used to be good at rescuing situations and giving hope to lost causes? Where did that skill go? And who wants to touch a man who has a relationship with death at centre stage?*

There have been two positive events in these last few days. First, as the handmade design of both of our bathrooms demonstrates, in the right mood Margarita can do some cool paintings,

---

* Margarita: 'The quality of our relationship changed. The trauma that entered our lives became a wall. I waited, but also needed very much to talk to you, to confront our mutual experience, the big fears. But there was only silence. When we went once to a couples' therapist, you explained you were trying to make peace with Death, and had no need for help. You suggested I needed support. And that was it.'

so I had been asking her for a long while to start creating something for the entire floor of our terrace. Recently, out of frustration I even started painting some coloured strips myself, with some of our leftover material.

Maybe it was my ridiculous doodles that forced her to start thinking about it properly. Eighty square metres can be quite overwhelming, but as we sat down and I drew five big, simple flowers on a piece of paper, it triggered something in her. She started conceptualizing that big space as a smaller garden for just a few flowers, and I now have the impression that she is going to start doing it. I can't take credit for the concept, but looking at a big problem as a small, feasible thing is helping us both in many ways.

The second positive aspect is that, regardless of which team is now supervising my pills, I will be spending some proper time with a group of women doctors, who seem very excited to start working on my experimental vaccine. It will involve being poked frequently with needles, but I will be hanging out with some women who are excited by my body – even if in a strange way. Fortunately, the main doctor for the vaccine gets along very well with my mother, and her younger assistants are even communicating with me via email, which is highly unusual in this hospital.

Usually, all communications are done via telephone or pieces of paper in an envelope. If they need to confirm one of my appointments, or have to move the date, all of that is done by an assistant (usually the voice of an old woman who has offered to do this kind of thing for the department), telling me something on the phone without even knowing what she's talking about. I can't wait to spend some time with those vaccine ladies.

Public health, here in Italy, is great in being universal and 'free', but it does require a lot of patience and hard work. Since I seem to be emotionally unable to distract myself with my old profession, I have begun taking an interest in all the experimental research groups in the hospital.

I remember visiting Milan during a summer break from university in the early nineties, and while my dad and I walked around the centre of town, crossing the little streets with those beautiful old-fashioned tramlines, we arrived at a fantastic modernist sculpture, in front of a church on a quiet pedestrian square.

He told me, 'You know Uncle Fabrizio, you know about his life here in Milan with all the homosexual crowd. Well, you also know that his friend had AIDS, and now . . . you know . . . Fabrizio has it as well.'

It wasn't easy for my father to tell me this. And in fact, I think he must have planned that walk and those locations to create a certain calmness in his delivery of this shocking news.

While back in the eighties I was aware that many artists and journalists had become involved publicly with AIDS, the stigma overwhelmed the reality. Somehow, even though I'd spent a whole summer at Uncle Fabrizio's house learning photography from the very best, and had occasionally even walked into drugged-up gatherings with his friends, I had never thought of him getting that illness. At the time, it was the social equivalent of having the plague.

At that time, there was no realistic cure on the market, but Fabrizio managed to get into one of the first experimental trials there in Milan, where he was living, and now he is almost sixty-five – still a pain in the arse – and will surely outlive us all. He had the right doctor, who helped him to catch the right boat, which was exploring the right seas in the right way, and completely sneaked out of that war. That does not mean that his conflicts with illness have not continued, but at least he is alive.

From the moment I started telling Miro, when I was dropping him off at kindergarten, that Daddy has to go to work, I have started to put on my more professional shirts, which allow me to treat my illness as a proper job. Perhaps it is desperate to conceive of myself walking through different hospital offices, doctors' rooms and clinical researchers' sections as being a professional human being. But unless you are a train or metro driver, or you happen to be Santa Claus, for my four-year-old child, work is something that is part of a narrative, where Mummy and Daddy go and do something that is similar to what he does in his kindergarten.

In any case, each morning I still tell him that Daddy has to go to work, so he can't stay at home and play with him. He has to go to school and I go to work. We will see each other and play at four, when I pick him up.

Being with a four-year-old is beautiful – it's fun and it challenges me in so many different ways – but even if a part of me would like to spend all my time with him in that little park surrounded by trains, I am unable to do so. I don't have the patience, I need to work, I need to find a way to bring peace to my battle with the Aliens, or to dispel from my head the continuous doubts and ridiculous statistics.

What I am slowly coming to terms with is that my reading is not coming back and I will have to continue telling Miro goodnight stories as I make them up on the go. I think of the events that have happened to him during the day and reorganize them as stories of animals or kids whose adventures can surprise my little boy and let him sleep in peace. Maybe it is this narrative-stretching exercise that has been helping me find the energy to undertake this impossible book project.

Or perhaps I need to focus the few energies that I have on another project, like finding a job which is properly remunerated and, through that, help my relationship with my wife. Something that can take me out of the house and let me come back in the evening with some tangible return on my time and investment. Buying flowers every time I go to the market no longer has any effect on Margarita. I don't think I do it because my father, Gastone, always filled our house with flowers.

I do not, and cannot, give up this battle.

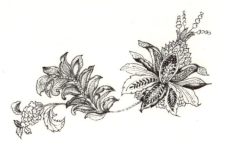

14

Love in an Indian Jungle

Rome and Jaipur, India, 2010

One day in 2010 the doorbell rang and the postman asked me courteously to come down from our top-floor apartment to sign off a document. Usually, the arrival of such letters reminds me that I should get a proper job, which could get our bills paid with less stress, or perhaps bring in the same amount only with fewer trips abroad, but this time we received a beautiful-looking letter that immediately brought joy to my heart.

For more than a month I had been keeping my trips to

London and Munich to a minimum, in order to stay close to my wife and take care of our son while she was visiting hospitals in Rome with her parents. For on top of having a frustrating time working at the Policlinico, Margarita was now having to help her parents, who had moved nearby, to deal with the Italian doctors who were trying to cure her father's pancreatic cancer.

Sadly, though, the tension between us had been rising. While being one of the bosses of my own production company did allow me some freedom, the frustration of not physically participating in the discussions with my partners and writers was becoming more obvious, as was Margarita's stress from the management of her parents.

So I presented that thick piece of paper to her theatrically, bending down on my knees, as if she were the Queen. Opening that envelope made her happier than I had seen her in years. The thick paper was cut in the shape of a hand and covered with Indian tattoos, and attached to the wedding finger there was a real ring. It was an invitation to Russell Brand and Katy Perry's wedding at the Aman-i-Khas resort, near Jaipur in Northern India. Neither Margarita nor I had ever been invited to a star-studded event like this before and even the design of the card made us excited.

A few weeks later, Katy and Russell sent us a lovely DVD package, with a series of self-shot clips of the two of them travelling romantically through India. Right at the beginning, after the image of the Taj Mahal, Katy says looking straight to the camera, 'Russell is about to eat gold!' to which he replies, 'While the world is about to collapse due to decline and fifty per cent of the world population is living on less than one dollar a day, we are here eating gold, real gold for dinner.' On our invitation, the text told the guests that rather than giving presents, we should contribute to a series of charities.

I had never been to India before and, besides some meetings and dinners with a few beautiful Indian actresses and charming producers during the Cannes Film Festival, I had never truly had any contact with their world. The generic details that we had from the wedding planners described an animal resort in the middle of the woods, somewhere near Jaipur. Last time I had met Katy in London, she had mentioned that the trip was rather draining and that while from Europe the flight was going to be eighteen hours, from LA it could take twenty-two hours, and after that we would all have to take a four-hour bus drive.

We had to wait a bit longer than expected for our visas because, as we learned, 'new' Italian citizens are treated 'differently' from 'true-blooded' ones. Finally, the visas were in our hands, we checked, and no vaccinations were necessary but Margarita, just to be sure, packed a large box of medicine to cover any possible emergency. Excitement was in the air. Her parents were well prepped for babysitting our two-year-old and in two weeks, we were going to be on a flight to London and then to India. The American organizers had told us that the whole event was going to be casual, apart from one of the nights when they would provide us with our attire, which all sounded cool. Then, at the last moment, came the instructions for the wedding day celebration. The dress for the day had to be 'White and Gold'.

This little piece of information destroyed weeks of work for Margarita, and for most of the other women who had been creating and choosing the right tone for the event. By chance, I found a gold jacket that fit me in a second-hand shop, but that did not resolve the main problem. At home that evening, disheartened and frustrated, Margarita pulled out a piece of material from the cupboard. And then another. And another. She and Jasmina got to work and until the day of departure our house became a fashion studio. They took a golden waistcoat from the 1800s, which was more an antique work of art than a piece of clothing. They flipped it on its head and sewed it on to her own white wedding dress. Then they covered it all with another golden fabric and *voilà* . . . we needed a bigger suitcase.

~

Even if the seats of our bus were comfortable, our four-hour drive on the Indian 'highways', with Matt Morgan, his new wife Katy, and Mister G and his wife, reminded us all of the fragility of life and importance of prayer. After a while listening to the trucks continuously sounding their horns, trying to overtake each other on those tiny roads, I made peace with my imminent death, feeling as if I was engaged in one of those Stockhausen concerts that my father used to listen to while he was cooking.

Night had fallen by the time we arrived, with the type of darkness that you only see when you are in the middle of nature. We sat down exhausted to eat some fantastic Indian food, surrounded by old-fashioned lanterns, then we were chaperoned by a military-looking man to our tent. I have crossed most of Europe camping, but even I had never seen such a cool tent before. It had an inbuilt stone shower and bath and right outside our 'door' there was a table and two comfortable leather chairs.

In the morning, while Margarita took time to prepare herself, I looked out into this wonder of trees, plants and flowers and I smiled. The soundscape was an entire opera performed by birds that I had never encountered before. Breathing out a stream of smoke from my first cigarette of the day, I felt stupefied by this experience and the world that my crazy friend Russell had brought us into.

In every corner there was an Indian servant standing with a gun slung around his shoulder. Upon our arrival, I had asked the British girl who was managing our 'hotel' why these men were all carrying guns, and she had told me that they were there to protect us, not from paparazzi but from the animals. This was, after all, the animals' world, not ours.

As I greeted one servant standing nearby and asked him where I could find some breakfast, he accompanied me the whole way out there, waited to see if I looked happy, and without saying a word walked back with his gun to his position near our tent. I walked towards a group of men who looked more or less my age. We chatted about the interminable trip we'd all had from different parts of the world, and even though the journey had been traumatic for all of us, we agreed that this location was quickly making us forget about it – as Katy had promised us it would.

There were three different 'tent' areas: one for Katy, Russell and their closest family, and two others where the various other friends were staying. Near our tent we had Matt and his wife Katy, then Russell's manager Nik Linnen and his dad John, and at the end of our row Trina and Adam Venit, who Russell explained to me was his new LA agent.

I'm sure that I have mentioned them earlier, as they are on the list of people who I credit with saving my life. No matter what the scientists might say, for me, it is all about the funda-mental human relationships with my characters, like the Italian-American nurse in Bethesda, or the young surgeon that operated on me in LA, who all have equal parts in my private superhero series.

That night we all dressed up in our casual wear and met in front of the big swimming pool, where the space had been completely reorganized to create a theatre stage. All the walk-ways throughout the entire park had been filled with beautifully arranged Indian flowers, but the most remarkable thing of all for me was to see Margarita leaving all her fears of wild animals behind and walking through the high grass looking and touching everything.

We ate a fantastic Indian dinner, the alcohol was flowing and the conversations bloomed. From the moment of our arrival, we all disregarded the fact that we had a pop star amongst us.

I moved around to meet some of Katy's group and immedi-ately ran into a man who told me he was going to conduct the ceremony. It took me a little while to get used to this character, as American preachers often look quite a bit different from my

Italian idea of priests standing in a church. I told him with a smile that Russell had been the priest at my wedding, expecting him to ask me some questions and maybe laugh about it, but his body tensed up, and he made sure to interrupt any further comment that I tried to make. He didn't understand or agree and wasn't even curious about the idea that Russell could have married us.

Unabashed, to improve the mood, I tried to throw some relativism into the conversation: 'You know, different cultures have different rituals. And I do like to play with more modern versions of—'

He shut me down again: 'There is only one Holy God, and that is the one that I carry with me.'

At that point, I retreated awkwardly towards the alcoholic drinks and told Margarita of this encounter. She calmed me down by bringing me into the discussion she was having with Trina and Amanda Fairey, who were also talking with David Baddiel and his wife Morwenna Banks, both great comedians in the UK, and together they quickly brought me back into our fun headspace.

I chatted with David about the last comedy film he had written, *The Infidel,* which is about an Islamic man who discovers that he is actually a Jew, and whose title was inspired by a short film that I had recently produced. The 2 Many Executives' version of *Infidel* was also a comedy, but about having dinner with a holocaust denier. At that point I told him of my encounter with the American priest, and, as it turned out, he had also run into him, and seemed even more shocked than I was. We started to think of what we could do about this, and the question was: 'Should we tell Russell?'

Baddiel and I discussed this issue further as the alcohol unleashed our emotions, and we decided that since we were both well acquainted with Russell, we had to assume that he already knew about this guy. The fact that he accepted the politics of this man and allowed him to be his priest was the ultimate proof of his love for Katy. No other person could bring him to accept something so radically different from his own belief system. In his world, such abominations of logic would be destroyed immediately with attacks of lucid comedy. This was acceptance. This was true love. This was the proof that Russell was ready to embrace a new, more difficult reality, and to change for this woman. I drank some more with Margarita, Matt and his wife, then we danced our way home through the dark paths of the forest without thinking of any possible strange animals.

We fell asleep immediately and easily, or so I thought. It could have been jet lag or the power of the drinks, but after all those intense religious discussions, something happened in my head. It was God; somehow he had decided to enter my dreams. I heard his voice say, 'Martino, calm down.'

To which I replied, 'Don't worry about me. If I'm still hearing your voice, I must still be drunk.'

'I understand what you're saying, as I am always drunk myself.'

As a sort of a wisecrack, I asked him, 'What do you take? What do you drink?'

To which, in all earnestness, he replied, 'Your love for me is my drug and my drink.'

'So why are you here in India?' I asked him.

'Why is anyone anywhere? I am always with you.'

'But then,' I asked impulsively, 'what's up with that priest that we met tonight? Why is he here creating stress in the midst of such harmony?'

'He is a lost soul. He arrived in a land of great love and faith and brought acrimony with him. Only hand luggage is allowed on this flight and he brought too many bags with him.'

'It is strange for me as well, but he is a Christian priest,' I said.

'Christians are no better than anyone else. Five thousand years before Jesus came down to save some of you, in this neck of the woods they were already praying for God Almighty.'

'That old? That's ancient,' I said.

'Hinduism is my biggest seller around here, but Buddhism, Jainism and Sikhism are also good niche markets.'

'You mean I can choose any religion and you will always be there to support me?' I asked.

'Sure,' he replied, 'I am here specifically for you. I know you need help and have opened up to me. And here I am.'

'Did I call you?' I asked, confused. 'I thought I was just a bit drunk.'

'Just know that I am here for you. And don't be angry about those who have lost themselves. Have patience and when you hit your head on a wall, do continue to believe, as I will be there for you.'

'Sure, God Almighty, or however is the best way to call you.'

At this point he said goodbye with a last adjuration: 'Be good to yourself and others.' And vanished in a dream.

The next morning we all woke up a bit dazed. Together with Matt and his wife, we asked for a driver to take us to the nearest town. We had been told by the organizers that upon exiting and entering the grounds, we would encounter a crew of paparazzi who had settled right outside. We set off in a jeep with our driver and his gun, and as the truck blocking the end of the road moved away, we left the excited paparazzi behind us and started looking at the trees full of monkeys, who seemed happy to see us.

It took us about fifteen minutes to drive to the closest town, where we stopped and took a walk and quickly discovered that just around the corner, there were three other jeeps with other members of our party. Katy Perry's father, also a preacher, was there and as we walked around together, I was delighted to see that, unlike the arrogant human of the night before, he was a charming man. We chatted easily, commenting on how strange it was for us to be in that town, which was so poor that it made us all feel awkward. The children smiled at us without asking for money, contrary to what I had been expecting. We gave them some pens and they smiled at us as we carried on our way. Not knowing how to deal with the fact that the world right outside our VIP park was so radically different, we went back, took a nap and then I jumped into our pool.

As I swam, feeling at peace with the plants all around, I spotted a man who Russell had told me I should definitely meet, because, as he said, we were from similar worlds. It was the American graffiti artist Shepard Fairey. While I was still in the water, and he was on the side wearing his jeans and Ramones T-shirt, I approached him and we started talking. We began with our admiration of this fantastic trip, and within less than a minute our discussion turned to art, politics and geography. When he started telling me about the project that he had recently done with Russell for the *Happiness* documentary, I immediately understood why Russell wanted us to meet.

Shepard and Russell had opened a shop in one of the big LA shopping malls, in which money was not accepted. People could come in and swap objects, books or socks for other objects. The big question was: 'What does it mean to have commerce without money?' It was great to feel that Russell had found his new world in that extraordinary city, together with his love for Katy. I could never have guessed that, quicker than a cheetah could pounce on a limping Berlusconi, Los Angeles was going to become, for me and my extended family, our new home.

Even though Margarita had allowed an ample amount of time to get dressed for the wedding, the golden-and-white construction that she had organized with her mother in Rome required a bit of assistance from me and, as usual, we ended up being the last people to leave our camp. We took one last picture, put the camera away and slipped into the fancy car that had been waiting to take us from one side of the park to the other.

Katy and Russell had not given any company or newspaper the permission to photograph their wedding. In fact, since we'd arrived, a team of American security guards had been constantly checking the perimeter of the property for possible entry points. But as we were the last people coming out, the paparazzi that had broken into the first layer of security went properly crazy, with their cameras pointed in our windows.

After their arrival at the wedding ceremony wearing traditional Indian clothes, Katy and Russell walked hand in hand amidst the heartfelt applause of all their guests. We were saluting them, their love, and all their work for bringing us on such an extraordinary adventure. No film and no set, no crowd or public acclamation could compare to this moment.

It doesn't feel right to tell you any more about their private wedding day, so I will leave it there as Classified Information.

The day after the wedding Katy turned twenty-six, and as it would have been impossible to equal the celebration of the night before, she organized a fantastically calm gathering when we all could relax. The whole time I had been looking for the right moment to talk to her, and as I saw Katy there with Russell, I approached and said to her, 'Thank you very much for having married my friend. I'm surprised, proud and almost in tears at seeing how happy you've made him. Already in the little time you've been together, you've changed him for the better in ways that I could never imagine.' And we hugged.

The next morning was wholly dedicated to goodbyes as everyone left at different times. While we were all hugging and taking pictures, Nik Linnen asked me to follow him and have a chat in the resort with Russell.

There, in the middle of India, accompanied by monkeys and sweeping birds, Russell stopped, stared straight into my eyes and said, 'Come to Los Angeles – we'll create big films and make the revolution there.'

And with that repetition of the beginning of Chapter Three, that's it, that's the end of the story as I've been writing it, and living it in the past tense, of the Hollywood dream that never happened, the *Bad Father* that never got made, and all my other beautiful tales.

I no longer know how one can construct a happy ending, but since that only happens in a certain type of Hollywood film and that reality is now well outside my health-care parameter, I can try to write the artful film that I've always wanted to create. The one where the drama leads the narration even when the comedy seems to be covering all the space, and where the good guys like me are also bad, and the bad characters deeply human.

Alex, let's just suck it in and keep going. I feel that there is a light at the end of this tunnel . . . or is it just a rainbow that I see out there?

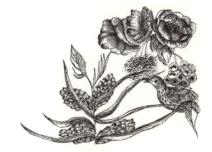

15

Alex and Me

Rome and Siena, 2011–12

Five years ago, when this book was just a chaos of notes and emails to myself, I wandered through the hospital in Rome where they had cut up my brain, searching for some clarification of my various handicaps. How long will it take for them to heal? What must I do to fix them? Who can make them disappear? And . . . when will I start reading again?

Fortunately, one day I arrived in a little room on the basement floor, where I met a proper human being with all the beautiful nooks and crannies of our species. She is a lovely speech-therapist lady with curly white hair and slightly crooked teeth, whose name I have tried to recall many times, but it keeps disappearing from my mind. Her good humour and constant curiosity about my strangeness gave me encouragement every time I arrived.

Her primary job is to help people who have had a stroke to retrain their brains. I've often found myself recalling the exact moment, at the end of our sixth meeting, when she told me the answer to my most urgent query: 'What is actually going on with my reading . . . and what can I do to re-learn it?'

Her eyes, behind her thick metal-rimmed glasses, conveyed a clear sense of regret. 'Due to the rather large excision in the left hemisphere of your brain, you now have five different and separate "issues" that do not allow you to read text.' Upon hearing that number, I smiled wryly and my left hand opened wide.

I will need to ask you for some patience as I attempt to summarize her explanation of those five issues. The first one is my problem with my short-term memory. Like most people, it was quite usual for me to stop briefly when I was typing, and while searching for the right word, discover a piece of text that brought me much more than the end of the sentence. During that little pause, the beginning of a new idea, or a new concept, could often be found.

Now, as soon as I return to the phrase after that short break, I realize that I have no recollection of what I had written, both at the beginning of that sentence and all the ones before. So I have to ask Alex to re-read me everything from the top. For example, he has read me this particularly long-winded section ninety-six times. After working on one single piece for so long, I then have to ask Alex to read me the entire chapter again, to remind me of the significance of that particular sentence, and how it should be followed.

For the second issue that I have to confront, I will start with a game. I'm sure you will have encountered the experiments with scrambled text, where the middle of words are all mixed up and only the first and last letters stay put, and yet you can read it all with no problem. 'The olny iprmoatnt tihng is taht the frist and lsat ltteer be at the rghit pclae.' Your reading is based on your recollection of the entire structure of that sentence.

The problem for me is that I have no recollection of what those words could be, and Alex's voice just reads it as the gobbledygook that it is, which is also how he constantly reads me my spelling mistakes, leaving me wondering, 'What was I trying to say with that sequence of letters?'

The third issue that confronts my new relationship with text is that, while reading, my eyes see only three letters at a time. As what happens on the right side of the brain affects the left side of the body, the big hole on the left side of my head has shortened the field of vision of my right eye. Which means that a good part of the text on the right side of a longer word simply disappears. This also doesn't allow me to see if there are any other words in that sentence. It's hard to do the necessary guessing game without that perspective.

The fourth and fifth issues that accompany me in the literary world every day . . . well, I'm sure they're just as relevant and powerfully stress-inducing as the others, but right now I don't remember them, which is a shame. What is even worse, though, is that shortly after I'd heard this rather scientific explanation from my therapist, I took a trip to London to earn some money and along the way missed three meetings with her. When I came back to Italy, I noticed that her phone number had disappeared from my ancient little Nokia, and it was also no longer pasted on the door of her office. After asking around the hospital, someone told me that she had turned sixty-five and retired.

As I tried to conceptualize the mixture of all five of those problems that she had worked on for me, and realized that I had managed to make even her character disappear, I found little trickles of human water falling down my face. This was going to be the incessant reality of my everyday life. And this is the reason why meditating has become essential for me. It allows me not to throw glasses or computers continuously against the walls.

To follow that rather tragic piece of storytelling, let me explain briefly my relationship with the beautiful male voice that accompanies me every step of the way. Thanks to my sister, the arrival on my computer of this text-to-speech programme has meant that I now have some kind of access to the written word. The name 'Alex' is not my creation. But the fact that his voice is American and never changes its tone even minimally, has allowed me to detach that name from a rather more violent Alex that in my teenage years lived in a strange part of my brain. I refer to the main character in the Stanley Kubrick film *Clockwork Orange*. Which is great, because I do have to get Alex to read and re-read text so many times that, if he were Kubrick's character, by now I would be dead.

Alex makes every detail of this book possible, but at the same time he flattens every single word that I choose to express my experiences, reality and emotions. Alex doesn't – and actually cannot – put the stresses and intonations in the right places, as a human voice would, which makes the meaning of most passages of text very hard to grasp.

Imagine receiving a love letter. One that is full of details and memories of a magic moment. Where your partner's choice of words reminds you of their body. And every little bit of it, every word that has been carefully chosen to convey an extremely private emotion, is spoken to you by the type of voice that advises you, 'In three minutes, bear left, then continue straight.'

So, the next time that you find yourself listening to that Sat-Nav voice in your car and start complaining, remember that it's actually a recording of a human voice, and that Alex, who has to deal with a much more complex vocabulary, is a flatter, computerized version of it. And that machines, also, occasionally need some of your love.

~

After a seemingly endless amount of work with Alex I found an email I recently sent to my American friend Emily James. I just needed to remind myself of my 'human' communications (it has taken 20 minutes and Alex has had to read me these last two sentences about 39 times before I was at peace with them).

Email to Emily James in NYC

Hey Em,

I am here in Rome breathing deeply in . . . and . . . out, continuously dealing with my doctors, and I have often found myself thinking of the documentary that you did in your neighbourhood, and I still find it great. I know that it is really aggravating that those TV commissioners etc. . . . don't understand the importance of your beautiful little story.

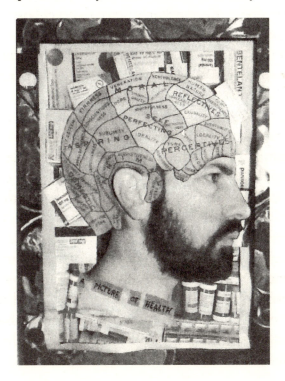

Maybe the new corporate investors, who are breaking down a city, step by step, shop after shop, and taking away the hard-working people from their life's investment, are so common that the public broadcasters don't see it as a 'worthwhile' history?

I guess we both know that, like it or not, this is the only boat we know how to drive, the only passion that we find relevant (and even if my ship has now more than a few gaps in its sails, I can't manage to make it stop).

Oh, yes . . . here is the big 'Job' that I have recently been working on. It's a way of working through my new relationships with the various boxes of pills that, I guess, have brought me to 'good health'.

Big hug and I hope to see you soon, Tino.

~

I'm in the office of the Sclavi company in Siena, one floor down from the Panificio Sclavi, the first shop that my grandfather and my grandmother set up in 1947. As the building is from the 1600s, expanding the work spaces from that architecture has been tricky. From the entrance of the shop there's a little set of stairs to a large room, where I used to play with the baker as a child and put the bread into the gigantic oven.

On the left, down a little walkway, there are a series of rooms with no windows where the sweets are made, and where I usually bring Miro to play when he's here. Making cakes and then bringing them home to show to Mum obviously gives Miro great satisfaction. The older man who works there smiles at me in exactly the same way as he did when I was a child.

Recently, due to the expansion of the company, Antonio has managed to find ways to increase the work space and I can visit some rooms that I had never seen before. Now, through another narrow passage, you enter a large room with lots of windows where a man (a bit younger than me) makes the various cornetti for the different shops and also for some of the bars in Siena. All these people start work at three or four o'clock in the morning.

Behind a metal door there are stairs that bring you to another dark room where the fresh pasta has always been made, and since those machines look identical to the ones I used to play with as a child, I point at them with a nostalgic smile, which causes the man working there to answer proudly, 'Yes, they're the original machines.' He has known me since he started to work here, when I was a teenager, so he shows me some of the more modern machines that he uses now.

The one that I really like squeezes all the air out of the plastic packaging of the pasta, allowing it to keep its freshness much longer. Traditionally, people would buy fresh pasta for the day they wanted to eat it, or at the latest the next day, but that's no longer the rhythm we all live in. We have to compete with the myriad of products available in the supermarkets, so a little bit of technological assistance is needed.

For a while I've been hearing from my uncle how badly the business of the bakeries is doing. I hope he understands that I'm here because I love him and that I'm offering him the few skills I still have, which could maybe contribute to making our company more economically viable.

Up the stairs and down the other side again is a little space where I always find myself having to bend my head down, as the roof seems to be too low for my big head. In fact, this is the head office of the Sclavi company. As usual, Antonio's desk is covered with papers and no computer. Hanging on the wall there are some well shot commercial photos of his face, partially covered by the wheat-flour with which he makes bread. I've never actually seen him make any of our products with his own hands, but then his central task is to run the whole company. And his refined sense of taste allows him to recognize a good batch of bread from a bad one.

I'm sitting beside his table counting money – the chore that Antonio or even my grandmother always made me do in the evenings at home after dinner. Like in the old days, with the constant background sound of a German police series on television, the various paper bags are opened, the receipts are pulled out and the money is counted. The aim is to compare the receipts of the bakery with the money that has been taken that day, and then put all the coins away. As a child, I was often given the coins that were left over from the accounts, which I would proudly bring to my room on the second floor. Who knows what happened to that stash of old Lire.

I ask the fifty-year-old account manager how I can connect to the Wi-Fi area and she tells me that they've not sorted it out yet. It seems that, even if all the different computers are on line, the man who comes to set up these things has not managed to fix the network properly. I look at the empty computer in front of me and ask if I can use it and the woman tells me that she doesn't know how it works.

She shows me that it has been put there with only one aim: to record the movements of the staff in all the ten shops. It does feel a bit scary sci-fi, but as money has gone missing in quite a few shops, I do accept that it is necessary. Pieces of bread are so small and light that it just takes a second, not entering the receipt, and the money is yours. If he allows me, I'm sure I can at least set up a proper internet presence for the company and do some web advertising: 'THE REAL BREAD . . . On the web!'

I've noticed that Antonio's belly seems to have become quite a bit larger than the last time that I looked at it a few years ago, while we wandered through the streets of DC in the spring. And his mood seems to fluctuate even quicker than usual. This morning, when we got into the office, he appeared interested and calm, reading through the paperwork in front of him, but as soon as one of his staff arrived and explained why the other letters weren't ready yet, his voice rose in annoyance, and I noticed that for all the people there it was almost as if his yelling was a normal part of their daily soundtrack in that little space.

'Come on! Let's just get it done. What are you waiting for? Come on, ****!'

Antonio's friend, assistant, colleague, boyfriend . . . anyway, he takes quite a bit of Antonio's yells, and somehow manages to reply occasionally, and explain, at the same volume, the reason why the material hasn't been prepared.

I take a tour with them around a few new shops that I've never seen before. In a huge supermarket some way outside the city, the Sclavi company now has a stand that Antonio has managed to set up, thanks to a good relationship. Every time he mentions his 'friendships', I end up thinking of his relationship with the Masons. Not that I really care, but while he's set up his younger boyfriend in the entrance level of that . . . club . . . I've never been offered such a thing. They wouldn't allow me to make a documentary about them, anyway.

The problem with all bakeries is that people no longer get food from the little shops; they pick it up in the supermarkets, where the prices are often lower. The concept of high-quality, fresh bread seems to be disappearing. The Sclavi company has always had the reputation in town of being more expensive than any other, but it has also been clear to most people that our quality is noticeably better. Antonio has always travelled to different bread fairs and he tries to stay on top of his industry. There was a long period during which he was the chief representative of all the Italian bread makers, a task that was primarily concerned with the laws specifying when the shops can be opened, and their relationship with the unions.

At the end of the day, while counting the money with his boyfriend and watching the usual German police TV series, I ask him how I can gradually start contributing to our company. I tell him of my thoughts about the website and how the market, especially the high-end market, is moving to the web.

When he explains to me that he doesn't have the money to pay me, I tell him that, as I presently have no money at all, and no hope of finding a job, I could work for very little. I would just go back and forth on a bus to Rome, or have Miro and Margarita come up to visit on the weekends. Still looking at the German policeman on the TV, he tells me, 'I'm used to my life, and I like to keep it as it is. For a few days, I'm happy to have you here. But after a while I'd find your presence annoying.'

He stops the discussion by ranting on about the economic crisis, that he hasn't found anyone to buy Villa Flora, and how expensive that house is to run. 'Just think of the monthly heating bills!' He goes on to tell me how much it cost him to lay off the husband of Asma, his cooking and cleaning lady. The guy had two wives, whom he beat, and was always more interested in his Islamic community than in his work . . . and so on . . . and so on.

~

I've had some bad news. I've received a letter from one of the institutional health care bodies saying that, from now on, I will be receiving only minimal monthly financial support.

Well, the story is this. After we had a meeting the other day with a doctor here in Rome for my statutory check-up, Margarita told me that I hadn't played my role well. I hadn't given them the impression that I was truly handicapped. Now with that letter in my hand, she has been proven right. While I will continue receiving a minimum monthly fee from the Italian state, similar to the amount that very old people get, there will no longer be any contribution for someone to help me manage my life, which was one of the primary sources of income for us. I guess they've decided that I can manage alone.

Margarita is right: there must be a less 'charming' version of myself that I could have used. But the woman doctor who checked up on me and read my various blood and MRI results, and made me walk back and forth with my one eye open, was already in conflict with Margarita when we walked in. Two women doctors in a small room have the potential to spark fire. And I just told her the truth . . . my main frustration is that the world around me has no way to recognize my handicaps.

I spend a lot of time waiting in queues with other handi-capped people, and I'm really happy that all of my body is still working properly. I can walk, jump, talk, hear . . . It's just the gap in my brain, which by itself is difficult to explain. In a city where everyone seems to expect a certain level of 'normal' trickery – where not giving receipts helps both the buyer and the seller – expressing the unnecessary details of a more sophisticated 'truth' is, in fact, just stupid.

Anyway, there's not much I can do about it now. I'll have to find a company that will give me enough to pay the mortgage and accept me and my whole crew of hidden handicaps, while at the same time keeping calm and not travelling too much.

~

It might seem as if I'm distracting myself with this project at a time when there are much higher stakes that I should focus on. How can I explain it to you and make you realize that this text is my doctor, and that I have to keep all these characters – Alex, the Aliens, my son, my wife, sister and mother – all rolling down these pages?

Otherwise I'll just be the next character in someone else's book, maybe the one who only exists in occasional flashbacks. I've already done all my historical scenes for this story and now I can only focus on my life as I am living it.

In fact, every step I take that brings me further away from that eighteen-month life expectancy gives this story extra . . . for the moment let me call it gravitas. I know that finding a way to earn some money would help me to confront the issues with life and my wife, and I do keep trying to do that but, at the same time, this meditative project with Alex will hopefully help at some point, or be useful for other people who find themselves in a situation where numbers are against them, and hopes are disappearing.

At the end of this stressful day, I finally got Alex to re-read me everything in this last chapter, and somehow I feel good, as if I actually achieved something. And that is pretty important – to bring some excitement into a world where my occasional encounters with my son's voice are the only positive narration.

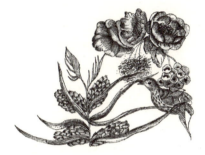

16

Back in the USA

New York, 2012

I've just arrived in America! I flew to DC two days ago to check in with Professor Fine, and to hear what he has got to say about the most recent developments in my brain and my use of the drug Temodal. I stayed at Adrian's new house which he and his new wife, who is an architect, are rebuilding. I had a lovely dinner with them and Ady's mother, whom I had met a few times when I was a kid in college. I actually recall having stayed at her house for a few weeks in 1992 while recording an album with my band, Shazzam, together with Ady's older brother, Jan-Nicolas.

His mother is a fantastic artist, who mostly paints seasonal flowers and has dedicated a good part of her life to teaching art in high schools. She came through her own battle with breast cancer a few years ago, and is one of those people with whom I really appreciated talking about this experience. It's the kind of discussion that I often try to avoid. During dinners or drinks, I usually give a quick synopsis of my situation and then try to find the most efficient way into a different subject, where I am not centre stage.

There are a few websites that are dedicated to brain cancer, in all its different interpretations, and occasionally Alex and I try to go through some of the less dramatic posts, but after about five minutes I usually shut off the sites and open up YouTube, to see some interviews with more optimistic, or at least cheerful characters – especially comedians.

On this particular evening, it was Adrian who moved the conversation on from our delicious fish to memories of when I was there for the radiotherapy sessions. He had interviewed me a few times and shot some interesting footage while we were walking along the memorial to the fallen in Vietnam and the Second World War.

I remember now that our original idea was to start filming parts of my life with the Aliens as it developed. That project has now moved on to a more pragmatic level, with my writing, but I wouldn't mind looking at those interviews, which reveal the way I conceived reality during that stage in my life. How could I have been so cheery and curious in that situation?

The team in Bethesda compared their new MRIs and the last one that I'd sent them from Rome and they seemed relaxed. Although they always appear interested in my battle, I can never get a proper opinion or advice out of them. I suppose that so long as they don't see any new Aliens wandering around in my head, they can't really offer alternatives to what I'm doing already in Rome.

Bianca thinks the reason they don't have anything to say is that they're actually a bit pissed off that I had a second operation, which erased a major part of the work I had done with them. Nevertheless, considering the financial and physical effort I've made to come and see them, I expected them to present me with some magic information, or at least a piece of advice about diet or sports, which would somehow calm down my discussions with Neil Gaiman's Death.

So now, as I'm writing, I'm in an apartment in New York City, and what can I say? It's just fantastic. It's next door to the Greenwich Hotel, which I guess is near SoHo, or Tribeca. My memory of this town is not only confused by my gap, but the fact that this southern part of Manhattan has changed so radically in the past twenty years.

I've taken over Russell and Katy's New York pad. Russell was lovely and organized for me to stay here, and from what I understand they haven't used it very much, since she's been travelling with her band for over a year. She was already preparing for this world tour when I was there in LA, working on *Bad Father*. Now that I think about it, that was almost exactly a year ago. I remember having Thanksgiving Day with Tom, Russell, Katy and her whole family. We played cards and various other games.

God, yes, now I remember, we played a game that Katy really liked where you have to guess words that are being mimed by one member of your team, and another . . . yes, another where you have to read a long list of names, which I tried and tried, but could not do. I should have realized during that game that I wasn't reading the text quickly enough. But since neither Katy nor my team pointed out how badly I was playing, I didn't worry too much. I must have thought that . . . what did I actually think? As the Aliens were already there, organizing for their big attack, I was attributing it all to stress (the same way I did a month later, while trying to write the third act of that film).

Here I definitely have the peace and quiet necessary to write this darn book, or whatever it's going to be. Many people have told me that this is the primary thing I should be doing, but so far I've found only little slivers of time to give it any proper attention. I recognize the therapeutic potential of this story, but the frustration of not being able to read or to remember anything is driving me crazy. I'm sure that, in this idyllic apartment, I will at least be able to put down some material that I can send around to editors or other writers, to see if anyone can help me by giving me an assistant, a co-writer, or whatever they think could work.

I don't expect to earn a lot from this project, but as I am now just burning money, and no one can hire me, it can't be worse than this. I'm enjoying narrating this story while sitting in this two-and-a-half storey apartment, and I'm sure that I'll notice the difference in my writing when I'm back in my normal life. Having a terrace in Manhattan gives me a different perspective on the world. It's quite chilly here in December, but I should try to go up every day and look at the city from this unique viewpoint.

Yesterday, I spent the day up on 125th Street, cooking turkey with a Macedonian doctor whom I had met only briefly in Skopje a few years ago. He is an old friend of Margarita's father and lives here, teaching at NYU. Our man-to-man relationship was a bit awkward in the beginning, but I ended up treasuring that day with him. It is Thanksgiving and there are so many things that I should be thankful for.

After that day of discussions about Macedonia, being an émigré, and the good and bad parts of the US, I wrote Margarita an email, detailing how she should consider the option of coming to teach here, due to our friend's contacts at the university. I do attempt to send emails or Skype with her as often as possible, as I continuously ask myself, 'How's it going with

Margarita?' My battles with the Aliens have forced the two of us to be in the same place for unusually long periods. In fact, I don't think Margarita and I have ever spent so much time together in the same house. She didn't like my trips before this, but perhaps it was exactly those times apart that helped us to keep our relationship alive. One of the imperatives for this New York trip is for me to find some calm and leave some space for Margarita, and hopefully, through that we will be able to rediscover each other.

I was just writing about my college rock band Shazzam, and pop, the name of the singer popped back into my head: John Wray. It is really random how names and words do come back for a second into my brain and just as quickly disappear, leaving behind a vaguely confusing memory. In this case I had written it down on my iPod and then immediately called John, who arrived just half an hour later by bicycle from Brooklyn. Many of my friends, due to the new environmental and good-health philosophy, are using bicycles as their main means of transport and I do find it quite cool.

I saw two high-tech bikes lying in the apartment, but I don't think I could trust my brain to let me use them in this city without great anxiety (which is exactly what I'm trying to avoid). I'm still attempting to make peace with a body that may look 'normal' from the outside, but from my perspective is obviously not.

As I explained earlier, the vision from the corner of my right eye has been cut out during the operation, which means that I can't see if there's someone walking next to me from the right, so I really can't imagine riding a bicycle along Broadway, where the taxis seem to jump from one street to another. Fortunately, when I walk alone, even if I don't remember the name of any street, I can recognize the architecture of the buildings and so I allow myself to get lost.

John wrote *Lowboy*, one of the last books that I was allowed to read with my own eyes, so I asked him for a general lesson on how you should structure your life while you're writing. I was surprised to learn that calmness, one of my priorities in life, is in fact crucial for such literary endeavours. It took him more than four years to write his story of a young paranoid schizophrenic who needs to save the world. So, Alex, I guess that we're right on schedule.

These days, I'm spending a lot of time by myself, which is good. Writing is going to be a long, long process, and I walk around deliberately trying to get lost, so I can then force myself to read the signs and talk to people. Usually when I ask someone for directions – and I choose whom I stop carefully, as everyone in NY has things to do and places to go – they pull out their phone and type in the address that I'm looking for, then they show me the map that has appeared on screen and we try to make sense of Google's directions. I often find myself having to look towards road signs, even if I can't read them, to show the kind person next to me that I'm being active and not just stupidly relying on them.

I went to Williamsburg to meet Josh Fox, an old friend from my liberal arts college at Oberlin, who, somehow, I have managed to keep in touch with. He's one of those people that always had his own vision of the world and followed his instincts, uninterested in becoming famous or being rich.

He had played successfully with arthouse theatre and film, before he ran into a story that in many ways overwhelmed him, bringing him into the centre of mainstream media and even a nomination for the Oscars. One day, when he was offered money by a company that wanted to dig for oil at his family's house through fracking, he began the adventure with his film *Gasland*, which documented him discovering how that industry is destroying the environment.

Josh and I talked easily about everything from new music to the social relevance of working, and our romantic stories that kept us alive. Amongst all these various themes, he told me that HBO was offering him a documentary about the relationship between our social addiction to mobile phones and . . . yes . . . brain cancer. Strangely, neither of us found this to be a coincidence. It felt right and natural that our paths would meet, nineteen years later, and force us back together.

We talked and talked, and it felt as if we were still there, back in 1993 in his grubby old car, getting a flat tyre on the highway on the way back to school after the Christmas break, and being rescued by a very religious man who, for the good of Jesus Christ, had stopped to help us. The part that makes this event memorable was that, while that man was fixing the tyre, Josh had pulled out his steel-string guitar and played some great tunes to help the Good Samaritan and me finish the job.

I immediately sent a message to Margarita telling her that, even if it might sound a bit too spiritual, I am almost over-whelmed by the positive signs arriving my way in this city. I told her that we really, really should think about this together: 'The energy is great here and definitely no one would give a shit about you not being from this country. Come on, almost no one here is actually American. Anyway, our lovely Macedonian doc says that you don't have to retake your doctor's degree in order to teach at his university.'

Emily James just arrived! She has crowd-funded her new feature documentary *Just Do It!* and is now in town to present it to a few producers and distributors. It's great to see her in this different context. We have met in many different cities, but I don't remember if our paths ever crossed here.

This evening, while showing off my aubergine Parmigiana skills, I asked her to give me some advice, or perhaps propose an editor who could help Russell to finish off his *Happiness* documentary. While before it was a rags-to-riches story, with Russell realizing that happiness does not come with fame or money, and asking the audience to follow him on his explo-rations from prisons to meditation centres, now that his Hollywood career has not taken off as expected, it has become more difficult for him to tell us this story the way he intended.

I can't sleep. I put the bedding for Emily on the big couch in the living room and from my perspective on the floor above, since she is quite small and is sleeping in an eye-mask with a fish design, she looks like she is swimming peacefully through the Hudson River.

Talking about all this happiness has got my head buzzing with different trains of thought. I'm afraid that writing this book is not only a therapeutic exercise for me. While I'm working on it, this project is bringing me . . . something that could even be called happiness. I'm not sure, but in attempting to confront this illness by typing away on this computer, this machine that I have humanized as Alex, I feel that I am touching something that is quite meaningful.

What I have learned up to now is that if I want to embrace death creatively, I need to share it with others. And I have the sensation that by doing so, I am adding time to my own life. I am worried that this project will not be something that simply disappears once I type *The End*. This will continue being a priority for me – one that very sadly might even overwhelm my marital commitments.

The marriage vows are all about putting the happiness of the other person first. Yes, I remember that, and it is absolutely true, but the more I make peace with the word Cancer, and see the sadness of all those men and women that I encounter while sitting in the waiting room of the oncology department, the more I am discovering that I need to share my newly learned perspective on illness and death. I know that it might seem a bit 'socialist hippy', but given the high stakes, we could even help each other to transcend together.

This morning, while sitting down on her couch and reading the newspaper, Emily informed me that Katy Perry's tour is passing by NY in a few days. Wow . . . I immediately checked with Russell and he told me not to worry about the apartment, because she doesn't use it while she's working, as the building doesn't have a security person and the entrance is directly on to the street. She stays in hotels, where she can also be close to her crew.

I got in touch with Katy's assistant and organized tickets for Emily, my dear old friend China from university, and her boyfriend. I am sure it will be a fun evening out. I'll make sure to nap a lot during the day, so I have some energy in the evening.

Yeah! It was a great show, and it almost overwhelmed my expectations. It was a fantastic experience, in every sense, and even though her music is in a completely different stratosphere from what I normally listen to, it pulled me along in her world and made me dance and smile. During the whole show, there are dancers bouncing about the stage, and at every song, the set and lights change radically.

Let's talk briefly about the clothes, because I think she must have changed her costume about eight times during the set. In fact, as she was singing one of her ironic-feminist songs that have now become classics, the dancers kept moving past her, stripping a seemingly endless number of dresses off her as they went. The strangest thing is that during the show I realized I actually know most of her songs, and quite a few of them I wasn't even aware were hers. She has managed to embed her music in everyone's lives.

I waited for a while as the audience left, and when her assistant appeared, who I knew from India and LA, I took the chance to go down to Katy's dressing room and thank her for the invitation, the show and, of course, the hospitality in her lovely apartment. She was as beautiful as ever, and considering she had been dancing and singing for more than eighty minutes she seemed quite energized. She is, after all, quite a bit younger than me (she must be . . . twenty-seven now . . . and not forty-something), and shaking her body around is a crucial part of her profession.

She told me that she and the whole crew were going to a club that evening and invited me to join them, but I smiled and explained that, thanks to my new relationship with my pills, I usually go to sleep at ten. I thanked her for the invite nevertheless.

Before leaving, I held her hands for a little while and told her how happy her show had made me, and how impressed I was that she had managed to keep her relationship with my dear friend alive. I explained to her how hugely he'd changed since they'd been together, and how impressive that was. As she hadn't seen him during the darker parts of his life, she had to believe me on this.

She was still smiling, but during my speech her face tightened up slightly. I guess she didn't completely agree. I had obviously poked a sensitive spot, because her answer was something along the lines of, 'Yes, but I do believe he still needs to take some steps to make our relationship as man and wife work.' I kissed her and went off to see Emily and my friends outside the concert hall, where at some point they had been kicked out by the bouncers.

I have been thinking a lot about the documentary with Josh, and even if I try my hardest to make it work, I don't think I can do it. It would be such a fantastic present for me, to work on a project that only needs me to be myself. I could even use and share my handicaps with the public, which would give some kind of relevance to my battle against the Aliens, and maybe even inspire other ill people to take on their struggles with creativity. Sadly, though, I don't believe that a conflict with the mobile phone industry will bring me, or the world outside, any real benefit, as I have learned that there are a plethora of reasons for why people get brain cancer. I talked this through with Josh and he agreed, and we will just think of something else to do together.

~

Only a few weeks later, while I sat on the terrace with Margarita, she told me that there were articles in all the press about

Russell sending his wife their divorce papers. I did not believe it. I've always avoided that kind of magazine, as they always stretch the truth for their own benefit, and very often it's pure conjecture. Those journalists are simply doing their job, as they understand it, and that day they probably needed something to fill a gap in their page. I am sure that it is not true . . .

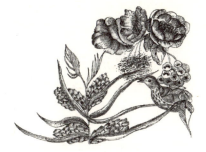

17

A Way to Fix Stressful Home Relations

Rome, Siena, 2012–13

Here is a list of all the good things in my life:

- Since I can't read the bills, those pieces of paper don't stress me any more.
- I don't have enough energy to go to parties and social events that I don't want to go to.
- I can't be attacked for going off and taking a nap.
- The Italian state gives me some money for my disability

- not much any more, but I'm still thankful for that – and for the fact that the government pays for my monthly packages of Temodal (my main drug), which cost 3,000 Euros.

- Margarita's car has a 'Disabled' sticker on it, which means that we can find parking anywhere, and she can drive through the centre of Rome, which is usually restricted to the residents.

- The economy seems to be focused on putting advertising in every corner of our life. Go ahead! Bombard me with all the glorious text you've got . . . I WON'T READ IT!

- These days I am really liking the people working on all these crazy, experimental, and perhaps revolutionary, medicines.

While working on my vaccine, I get to spend a lot of time with some truly beautiful, kind and hard-working female doctors and nurses. Every morning that I go in to see them, I walk in and feel there is hope in their movements and in their smiles.

I am learning that a research trial is judged by the number of research groups with humans it has assessed. This one is regarded quite seriously, as it is in its third stage. That means it has already been tested in three different ways, the third one being the last before it can be used in the open market. I assume that they have, at some point, tried it out on four-footed little animals.

Come on, Alex, let's pick it up . . . I'm getting into science and I need some help with the names . . . and not only of animals.

If it works, I'll have to look into where the vaccine ends up, as it has been partly financed by American and Italian hospitals and universities (Duke and Policlinico), and partly by some pharmaceutical companies. I wonder what the packaging of the product will look like. Before giving my blood and soul to this trial, can I ask them to put a clause in their contract that

I would like to have a link to my website somewhere in the credits? You know, that sheet of paper that always comes with those pills ;-).

I know that emoticons get Alex confused. In fact, they confuse me as well, but I find that I make them appear – and occasionally also go back and erase them – because I am unsure of the emotions that I am trying to convey. You know, Alex's voice is lovely, but it doesn't deliver any sense of my humanity. That is perhaps a whole other issue, that I will have to confront with my wife. Perhaps I am becoming less emotional. Can I really blame Alex?

~

This morning we all met about three minutes away from the Policlinico in a small, two-storey house, built in the 1870s, when Rome had left the Papacy and joined the new Italian nation state. There we met a young female doctor, who told us, 'In a few minutes we'll have a place for you. We're just setting it up.' She stopped briefly as if she had forgotten something, then went on, 'It will take three or four hours for us to take out what we need.'

I pointed towards a room with a long row of comfortable single couches and asked, 'Is this the place where I'll be under the needle for all that time?' She smiled apologetically and nodded her head.

This is an exciting project for them, because at the end of the day they will have only a few hours to mix my sample up with the brain tissue and get them to work together. They tell me that in nine days they'll be able to see if it really works, and then they will decide exactly when to call me in to re-inject my home-made vaccine.

Originally, this team was concentrating on woman's gynae-cological cancer, but as it emerged that this type of vaccine they were using also worked for brain cancers, they have now entered my beautiful world. They are encouraged by the results that both they and the Americans have been having so far, and as a team of women they generally have a different mood. Their squad is made up of a thirty-two-year-old doctor, a fifty-five-year-old professor, and their twenty-eight-year-old assistant. In order for me to be accepted as part of their project, I have already had to do a whole series of blood and breath tests, but those were easy.

Today the nurses will try to extract some of my bone-marrow cells that haven't yet matured into immune systems, and then they will take them to the doctors in their lab, who will sing them nice songs, tell them stories and generally treat them well, in order to nurture and so transform them into dendritic cells.

These dendritic cells are really important, because they are the ones that can learn to seek and destroy the Aliens in my head when exposed to the biomarkers, which are the parts of my brain that the surgeon handed them during my last operation. The reason why I am the one telling you this rather than the doctors is that when they speak about it sounds something like this:

The vaccine is composed of autologous mature dendritic cells pulsed with tumour lysate and a long peptide corresponding to EGFRvIII. We'll use the combination of both since Martino's tumour was positive for EGFRvIII antigen expression and we do not have enough tumour lysate. The plan is to terminate the DC injection schedule and utilize the peptide alone in a consolidation treatment.

While I'm sure that a few of you might find this explanation a compelling read, for me, listening to Alex's voice reading it to me for the thirty-seventh time, I am still confused. And it is all, at least in theory, about my own brain!

Here are my thoughts a few hours into the trial. Although the energy of all these women is great, I am currently feeling the pain. My veins are kind of sick of being cannulated continuously, and at the same time the chemo is draining out all their energy. The room is full of at least twenty other people being poked and prodded for their diverse illnesses, but those two young girls by the door, don't tell me they're sick – they can't be like me. They must be here for some other reason. They have been smiling my way empathetically.

I ask Margarita to find a nurse who can bring me something warm, like a blanket, because I am freezing. Is the temperature shift due to this back and forth of my blood? Why is it so difficult to ask someone else what they have? Fortunately, as the two girls leave the room with their big smiles, I hear the nurses talking to each other and I understand they're not sick; they were there to donate blood.

'I'm used to having a needle in my arm when I'm in hospital. It's fine, you get used to that. But this kind of experimental blood selection is more painful than usual, as they have to continuously withdraw my blood out of my vein, and then, once it is emptied of the material they need, put it back from another needle set up in my other arm. I'm really not liking this experience. I have now been here for the past three hours and I can't deal with it any longer.

The room is slowly emptying and I am trying not to groan too loudly, as a few lovely people are still here with something being injected through their veins, but why does it seem to be getting worse? That's not normal, is it? Margarita is sitting next to me reading something and replies to my discomfort with 'just a little bit more'. I understand that I'm being annoying, but come on, I've heard the 'little bit more' a few times already – did I not give them enough?

As soon as the nurse comes by, I smile ironically at her and ask if she can make it stop. She looks at the plastic bag full of a lightly red juice that has been pumping out of my blood, goes back to her room and returns nodding her head, as a sign of being satisfied. Margarita puts down her book and smiles at me when I start breathing a bit more calmly, and as the needles come out of my arms, I close my eyes and think of the trip that my red juice will have now. Someone is going to rush it to those ladies, who are going to work all night to make sure that it will hang out with my old Aliens, and teach them to believe that being part of a vaccine crew is much cooler for them and their progeny.

From what I understand, it will take them ten days before they know if all my bits are looking happy and the finished batch has been activated, and if so, they will freeze them and decide exactly when to re-inject the dendritic vaccine into my blood.

Right before leaving this room, which is now empty and being cleaned up, I think of this day with the nurses and those two girls, and know that I will come back here again, if at any point this institution will accept my blood as a donation to others. Everything about this place, from science to emotions, is important. Maybe it is the historical architecture, the lower ceiling of this clinic that has allowed me to feel detached from the big industrial complex of a hospital and bring me back to a dimension where everyone seems to care about how they are spending their lives.

In fact, while lying here today, I have decided to assist the work of the dendritic vaccine, and from now on I'll become a proper vegetarian, or at least a 'pescatarian', as some hippies that I know call it. It is just two steps away from being vegan.

～

I visited the clinic a week later to check on the development of my dendritic cells and sadly, they told me that they could not make it work. They will try it again, but that does mean I will need to come back to these ladies and redo the whole palaver from the beginning.

～

Two weeks ago, I was asked to offer my brain to a bunch of experimental researchers, because they need tumours like mine for their tests. This request came from a fifty-year-old doctor, who seemed quite normal, meaning that he appeared to be more like a 'dude' than the usual 'scientist' type. But as I talked to him about his project, it emerged that their study is only in the first round of tests, so at the moment it would have zero effect on my illness.

This did not make me feel enthusiastic, especially when they explained that in order to help them I would have to go to their clinic and get a forty-minute MRI, then as soon as I got on my feet they would bounce a metal stake near my brain for ten minutes. After that, to put a cherry on top, they then would lie me down again and do another MRI, to check the difference between before and after. Did I mention that they would have to do this for two days in a row?

In order for these researchers to save the world, they need people like me to take part in their experiments, so I agreed. The idea being that they could compare how my brain looked before and after it was banged around by their wooden stick. On average I now do an MRI every two months. Believe me, it's quite disturbing to have your head locked in a machine that yells very loud and unrhythmic sounds into your ears. But it's also quite funny to see these young doctors, who are collaborating with the Israeli Hospital, get so excited about doing this test on someone like me.

While they were looking at my old MRIs, I asked them if they had recognized that the big hole in the left side of my brain has been artfully created. With my finger on their computer screen I showed them how my gap is in the clear shape of a big bird standing with his head up, looking at the sky from the front of my face in the direction of my left eye, while his little feet are almost surrounded by his fat belly.

They looked back at me a bit confused, so I guess they had never thought of a hole in the brain in such terms. I explained to them that, as far as I know, our consciousness is simply something that science is not used to studying, and they are missing the true relationship between our material brains and our decidedly non-material minds. Perhaps I should introduce them to my Ned Flanders hypnotherapist and then they can appreciate how our minds can influence our physical self. Sadly, their emphatic belief in scans filters out the nuances of subjectivity.

I understand that for them I am a freak. I have no problem letting them believe that my 'strange' thoughts are due to the operation, whereas if they had met me a year before in a bar, they would probably have found my 'normal old self' much weirder.

Margarita and I had talked about this trial, and in part I had agreed because this group of researchers had found me through Ada Francia. Sadly, when Margarita set up the appointments, she did not think of the fact that after having repeated this whole 'bang bang' palaver for two days in a row, I would arrive at Miro's fifth birthday celebration, in the park with all the kids, completely physically and emotionally shattered. But since she did not want to compromise her relationship with Ada, that is what happened.

God, how stressful my life has become since I've had to live and think continuously of pharmaceuticals. First you get your head around the idea that, like it or not, you're going to die. That concept got into my head pretty quickly. How the rest of my world is going to cope with it is a more difficult one for me to confront. Everybody will encounter the concept of death sooner or later, but unless you have to tackle it fairly young, it remains abstract. My Uncle Antonio, who will be turning seventy soon and has had anal cancer for a while, does not even vaguely want to talk with me about death.

He has no children, so maybe he has the freedom to ignore it. As he says, 'I don't care what happens once I'm dead. I won't be there to worry about it.' Perhaps it is those mathematical predictions all over the internet about life expectancy with my condition that make me think of death as a clear concept, or at least as clear as one can have it.

The doctors that I have met up to now, here in the Policlinico, have been really clever in their management of my psychological development with this issue. I have never been led by any of the doctors, older, younger, surgeons or oncologists, into a discussion of my probable, or imminent, death. I guess they simply don't view it as a useful contribution. I am aware that I will undoubtedly die, and perhaps I am more aware of this universal inevitability than most other human beings in their early forties.

It took a bit of pushing from my side, but a few months ago, Margarita finally managed to set up some meetings with a psychiatrist. It is a world that undeniably belongs to my wife and only she could choose the doctor who might help us to resolve our marital crisis. I'm not sure, but it does feel as if coming in as a patient is a bit 'shameful' for her. In fact, that word itself is something with such a complex and deep-rooted legacy that, perhaps due to my illness, I've decided not to engage with it. Which might be a problem, since most people are driven by shame.

I remember that while studying, Margarita had to do some therapy herself as an exercise, and from her experience I understood that it could be intense. Since the very beginning of her courses here in Rome, I have been in tune with her school of thought. Amongst the myriad psycho-therapeutic philosophies, I find that the way she and her colleagues look at the world is refreshing. It is not because I am in love and married to her. Even on paper, it does seem to make sense. Like the German political philosophy that I appreciated during my studies, these psychiatrists seem to focus on pragmatic solutions, with an awareness of a wider narrative.

This type of psychiatry has one of those ridiculously long names that I will continue to have to look up on the internet, because I'm sure that in one minute it will have disappeared from my head. It is: Post-Rationalist Cognitive Therapy. And the most important theorist, whom I do remember from those old conversations, is Professor Guidano.

I am in no way capable of getting my mind into the complexity of these theories. When my brain was working, I already tended to lose bits of the broader philosophy, but as some of it is crucial to making sense of the wider story of my wife, the traumatic arrival of my oncological stakes and me, I'll give it my best try.

I have been cutting and re-pasting together old artistic photos that I took while living in Brixton, in the years after my father's death, and I recognize that I do that now because I can't read a book and I feel the need to put my brain in a different headspace, away from oncology or that lovely lady death. What I am learning is that by doing these exercises of sequencing events in images in scenes, I am re-interpreting them and assigning them all a narrative plot. Stay with me for a while, because I have just realized that this is actually the analysis of why and how I am writing this book that you are currently reading.

I understand that the possibility of death usually makes people more anxious if they feel they have not accomplished any positive task in the life that they are living, and so this book, like those artful designs, is confronting it directly.

OK, I've found a bit on the internet that talks about this kind of psychological theory much more clearly than I can, and it's not even too complicated (I really like it when theoretically complicated things are made simple):

It is inevitable in any person's life that unpredictable events occur each day and every moment. Any of these change our way of life, change our expectations and these events continue to be disturbing until we manage to integrate them in the history of our lives. For Guidano, the casual has been involved in the sequence of life events and at the same time the disturbing sense, which has been experienced when the unpredictable event occurred, has been transformed into a further tint from which to experiment the sense of continuity and of uniqueness of one's own life history.[*]

At the end of every session that we had with that psychiatrist, I think both Margarita and I felt cleansed. Even if I was 'obviously' the one who had to pay the bill, I didn't mind because, for days after, we didn't get into silly arguments or fights, so it was worth the expense. After a few months, the therapist asked us to do one-on-one sessions, which I tacitly understood as her need to confront our individual issues alone with her. During every meeting that I had with her we would always end up talking about my relationship with death. She really did have an extraordinary curiosity for that particular theme.

OK . . . the occasional discussion about death might be necessary for me, but certainly not for a better relationship with my wife. She winces whenever I mention that word, even when I try to package it as part of an obvious joke. I had pushed for us to do those meetings so that I could get some advice about managing our stressful relationship, and perhaps even find a way that I could explain to her how I still love her, even though my head is full of radically different, and sadly more important thoughts.[†]

During my meditative teachings in LA, I had learned that, even in its most profound meditative forms, consciousness does transcend the living body. And as death is a part of life that

---

[*] 'Narrative in Post-Rationalist Cognitive Therapy' by Alfredo Ruiz. Translated by Susana Aronsohn, Instituto de Terapia Cognitiva, Santiago, Chile, 1997.

[†] Margarita: 'I was really putting an effort into going out. One of those evenings I ran into a couple where the wife had just passed through breast cancer. Her husband told me of their detachment, both from the world outside and also from each other. The difficulties of a social life after something like that. The moments when you realize that those party people are only talking about discounts in a certain shop and you can either stand up and leave or . . . stop talking. And I did not even have the strength to laugh about it.'

has forced itself on to me, I try continuously to find interesting ways of making it relevant, by thinking of the people I will leave behind me and the way in which they will allow me to transcend. I really do dig it, but that is quite a tricky thought to have in your head while entering a party. Meditation helps me to sustain attention on a single object, while also helping me to be openly aware of the entire field of experience, without selecting or suppressing anything that arises. But when the world around me very obviously does not want, or is not ready to confront, what is in my thoughts . . . well, I would rather stay at home and put my son to bed.

During our wider discussions about meditation, my psychiatrist gave me the impression that she knew what I was talking about and, in fact, she told me that it could help me. I do not think that the ancient Asian Buddhist philosophies, on which part of my new vision of the world is now based, are so far away from these psychiatrists' more scientific concepts. Were it not for the continuous issues between modernity and religion, I could also imagine myself doing a faithful recitation of the rosary twice a day. I have not done it since I was a little boy, but I assume that reciting 150 Hail Marys has a similar rhythm that also cleanses all thoughts.

Finally, a few months later, the psychiatrist told me that from now on she was going to work only with Margarita and that I should find another doctor if I wanted to continue with this therapy. In their discipline, you can't go more than one and a half years with therapy and a therapist cannot follow two partners at the same time. As the idea from the beginning was for me to use an outside person to help us fix our marriage, and so that I could talk about death with someone for free . . . I just stopped going. I am still sad about not having asked her about Margarita's relationship with art, though. Her huge flowers, which she painted on our terrace, have been lying there for ages, half finished. What is that a sign of?

～

The other day, when I went out to do my shopping in the street market, I passed Rosi's bar. Next to a handicapped woman, who is always outside by the umbrellas looking a bit lost, I saw Rosi sitting down on a plastic chair with a big woollen hat on her head. As I got closer, I realized that both of her eyes were bruised from tiredness, and she didn't seem to have any hair.

While purchasing my green, yellow and red food, I thought about her, and no matter how many different narratives I created in my head, there was only one possible story. It was so obvious that I wanted to delete it. Rosi is undeniably under attack, and that is the violent truth.

Looking at my puffy face in the reflection of a shop window, I felt bonded with her. Since then, I have started to drop into her bar in the morning and get my freshly squeezed orange juice from them, even if it isn't nearly as good as the one from Necci. In the evening, when all the normal shops are shut, I pass by there and, although I know they only have full fat milk, I walk in and buy it.

I should find the right moment to have a chat with her. We could share war stories, and I could make her feel my empathy. Maybe we'll even end up having a laugh about it all. I haven't managed it yet, though, and I don't know why it is so difficult to talk about these things.

~

The fact that only two million people speak Macedonian, and it is professionally not too useful, should not have been an excuse for me not to learn the language. I should have done it because I love my wife and am interested in her history and in the world in which she has been raised. Now that I have difficulty finding words in any of my three languages, that mission has died completely, so I decided to put my energies into more artistic types of communication.

The first step for me is to censor myself from talking continuously about oncology and the tales of the Alien attacks in my head, as they always end up in a high-stakes battle between life and death. It took me a while, and probably a few scars on my lovely wife's heart, but I am learning that censorship is for the greater good.

So I substitute it with Art, as at least it's a language with which we have grown up together. OK, I no longer remember the names of any artists, or shows, or designers that we used to chat about in the evenings while smoking cigarettes and drinking red wine on the terrace, but it is visual. I can Google-image a few words and while scrolling through its pages, I know that at some point I will find the crucial name, style or movement that I was trying to contribute to our discussion.

Unfortunately, that does require a different rhythm to our conversation. A different kind of patience that I can't take for granted, especially when I interrupt Margarita from whatever she is reading, and she then has to wait three or four minutes before I can get Alex to read out information from a website that I thought she might be interested in. Usually, by that point, her mind is already somewhere else.

'You know, the main artist in New York in the 1980s . . . who came from advertising and helped us all look at advertising as art . . . You know . . . the images of single tins of soup . . . Yes, him . . .' What was the important part of that? Even after two minutes where through Google Alex read out loud 'everything you want to know about Andy Warhol soup'. It's still not that interesting, but for me it's an achievement, like a child taking their first step – but in contrast to that child, I know that it will take me exactly the same amount of time to re-find that same simple artistic name or concept. Why am I so proud of having said something obvious? It does not feel as if I am getting any better.

At times, I think the reason why we are not getting along is because I no longer smoke or drink. People do change quite radically when they put that kind of stuff in their mouth. Now that I am totally clean, I have noticed how it affects almost everyone in the morning before and after they inject coffee into their body. Moods change and as people experience that physical movement together, well, they share something together. Which is what we don't do.

We are close to our wedding anniversary and I've been working on a photo art book, telling the story of our relationship romantically, from the beginning to now. It is about seven pages full of images, which I have cut and pasted together. The fact that this project is forcing me to think constantly of the beautiful moments that I have lived with her, and of the joy I am sure this will bring her, makes me feel proud. Even if I am not feeling optimistic about relearning how to read, I do know, at least, that by putting an equivalent amount of effort into fixing our relationship, I will make this work.

By using art as a substitute for words, Margarita will be able to read my sincere emotions better. There is no voice in my computer that can help me with that type of communication, so I have to find other ways for us to read each other's feelings. Photoshop, like most other programmes, communicates with us by using long lists of words, so I have had to be artful even in my choice of software. Fortunately, while looking for interactive games for Miro, I have run into a few rather limited apps with which I can create something, which I have decided to accept as an artistic limitation.

Oops . . . but I guess it doesn't work like that. I'm not a therapist and I've just managed to get this totally wrong, like everything else I do. Due to the fact that I have been pissed off with her in the last week, she has now become pissed off at me. So when I finally found a calm moment to give her my artful photographic love story, she was feeling stressed and didn't show much interest in it. I really did think this was going to work. Now, those seven pages are just lying there on the couch, waiting for someone to unconsciously sit on them. I have a headache, and I need to take a nap.

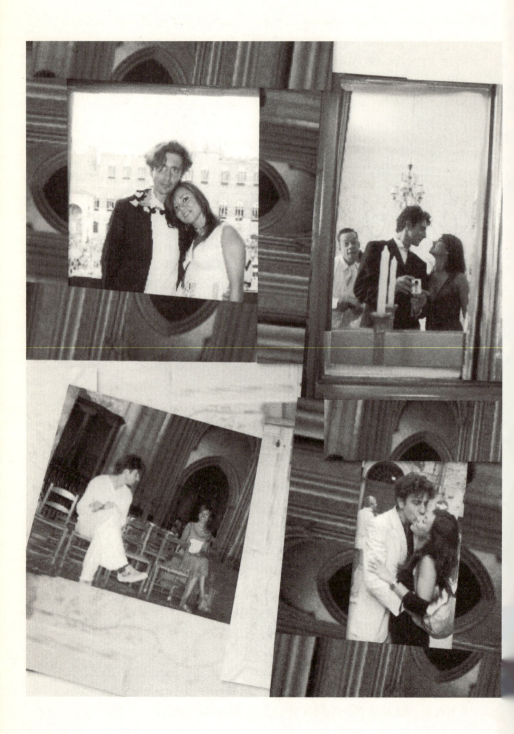

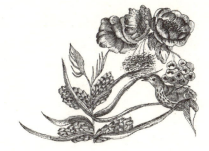

18

My Endless Affair with Difficult People

Rome, London, Munich, 2014

Email to Russell Brand in LA:

Hey Rus,

I hope all is well there in sunny land.

Since the lovely ladies that are working on my dendritic vaccine messed up the first batch, I had to give them another four hours of my blood the other day. Given how cool they are, I would lie down on their couch any time they want, but fortunately it appears they have now made a proper batch of it, and so . . . every two weeks I have to be in Rome for my dose of the dendritic vaccine.

I'll call you next week (when Miro is back to school post-chickenpox) and as soon as I am finished with these injections, I'll start to organize a trip up there to see you guys. I have to pass by DC anyway to see the docs there, so I'll arrange something around that.

In the meantime, I've got a little story that I think you'll like.

A few weeks ago, tired of my body being continuously injected with so many drugs and making peace with the fact that I'll most probably have to take Temodal, my main drug, for the rest of my life, I decided that I should at least get off cortisone – which I have always hated, as it makes my whole body puff up. So I did that, and even though I'm still fat, I have the feeling that I'll soon become a slightly prettier fat dude.

Yesterday it was really hot and to kick away my constant sleepiness, I set myself the task of fixing the taps in both bathrooms, as the water was simply not coming out properly. I assumed that it couldn't be too difficult, so I tried my best. Although I couldn't scratch or pull out the dirt in either of the bathrooms with my fingers, I saw there was a screwy bit right by the tap, which looked like it was made to be unscrewed. It felt like, you know . . . those jars of jam that have been closed for too long, and I thought that by pulling really hard, maybe with the bottom of my T-shirt in my hand, I could open it. I even tried putting some boiling water on it and then pulling, but nothing budged.

Margarita was up on the terrace with her magazines and I really wanted to show her I'm not an idiot. But I felt one of my headaches coming, so I took a nap, assuming that the taps would probably loosen up by themselves after sitting in the hot water for a while.

I woke up and tried again, but they still did not budge. So I went to the kitchen, picked up some big, strong scissors that have a bit in the bottom part, by the handles, that I could use to push together and unscrew them. Bang, bang, bang . . . like that classic story of the little kid who magically pulls out the sword from the . . . wherever it was stuck . . . I unscrewed both of them with no problem. I put them into a cup, immersed them in vinegar and finally detached the bits from the taps, which were in fact filled with debris. The water was flowing out happily and so was my mood.

I took my cup with my precious bits up the stairs to show Margarita my achievement and it kind of worked. I kept our conversation focused on the essentials, as there are quite a few other things that still need to be fixed, both on the terrace and below, but the wall between us was breaking down. We continued talking as we moved towards the stairs. I needed to finish off that job. Without wanting to interrupt her train of thought, I took my eyes off her for a second and started to walk down the stairway. I had been distracted by something, as though my eyes had caught the movement of a bird as it whizzed by.

Did I see something strange just because of the gap in my right eye? I walked down the stairs, and then turned left along the hallway, where I had seen that image from the terrace. It all looked normal as I stepped into the bedroom. Maybe I was letting my sick eyes fool me, but as I took one more step towards our closet . . . I froze. There was a man lying on the floor on the other side of our bed. Very slowly he pulled himself up and raised his hands over his head. The focus of his eyes made me realize that I was still carrying those large iron scissors in my right hand.

What is the probability that, walking through my own house, I would have violent-looking metal scissors in my hands? Mate, it was really amazing how at this stage my character changed radically and from that moment on, I was controlled completely by pure instinct. All the emotions of the past few months brought out my core male self. It is rare for any of us to encounter someone who is truly wrong, whose only aim is to steal your stuff. The tone of my voice rose, and so did my hand and the scissors. All kinds of words started pouring out of my mouth that I never knew were in my vocabulary.

While I hate my own body, which is all fat and puffed out due to the various pharmaceuticals, I realized that in this extreme encounter it had a very different and useful representation. I became conscious that the thief, who had been hiding under my marital bed, was now standing next to a very large, black-bearded man with an extremely loud voice, and very sharp-looking scissors in his hand.

I was not, and did not look like a sick person. Perhaps for the first time in my life, I was threatening. My words, my movements and my eyes were clearly those of a person who was close to death and now motivated to make this man suffer the same fear.

It must have been only a minute later that my confrontation with this thief crossed paths with my wife's character. It was a unique marital moment. Margarita's Macedonian emotions, which I had encountered in the past, now exploded into an extreme hatred.

Thanks to her emotional screaming, a few seconds after her arrival in my standoff, our whole neighbourhood was aware of what was happening. I assumed that between us two, and the sound now coming from outside the windows, he must have been quite overwhelmed. He was obviously a true professional, as with his hands raised like a lost man in front of a gun crew, he slowly walked his way backwards towards the door.

The days, weeks, months, the pressure and the fear of imminent death, and the destruction of my family life, all came together and focused on that set of scissors. Without pondering I pushed them through the belly of our unwelcome guest, of this torturer of private space, if any of it remained. His legs fell to the ground and his right eye received the blow of the scissors heading through the first section of his brain area. The brain does not have much sensation . . . I know . . . so I freely travelled through his skull with these metal kitchen implements.

The repercussions of this act could be many, but the feeling of that moment, the release and anxiety of my own death, finally came out. I was higher, stronger and more in control than the creature below my legs. The cancer, the medicines, the orders of the doctors. Alive or not, I was in control and I had finally found a character who had made, without any doubt, the wrong decision and unexpectedly for him, met the wrong cancer patient!

Our front door was still open from his entry and while walking slowly backwards, he stepped out. Protecting his head from the flight of our baby's bicycle, which my wife was using as her sword, he ran down the stairs and then walked very calmly out of the house door, in front of the various people who had come out to see what was happening after hearing my wife's yells.

After I had checked that Margarita was fine, I went down the stairs and saw that the people on the street didn't realize the man who had just walked out so casually was part of this whole drama. One would assume that a thief would run after such a confrontation, but as I came out I saw him strolling down the street. Still holding those metal scissors, I started screaming at him, and in my socks, I began to run after him. At that stage the street observers worked out who he was and they, too, started yelling.

Within a second he ran into a little side street, and I would never find him again.

I guess this was a strange way of temporarily fixing my marital conflicts.

Ciao, be good.

PS: Oh, yes. I finally got the first doses of my dendritic vaccine, but why do they really have to inject it right next to my penis?

~

I am walking away from our house, escaping from yet another row, when I see a packet of cigarettes on the ground. It looks almost full. After holding it in my hand for a minute, I put one in my mouth, look right and stop three African guys, who light it up for me, while continuing a conversation in their own language. It's the first one in three years.

I am making a call on my cheap little mobile phone, certain

that, after the usual sound of a foreign phone ringing, I'll hear a female computer voice say, 'Leave a message.' Wow! Russell actually answers. How is that possible? Very rarely does he pick up incoming calls, unless he is waiting for them to buzz. I am so glad, as I really need to hear his voice right now. I know that he, of all people, will understand my marital stress, and maybe even connect with my thoughts about a potential divorce. I have been trying my best to prioritize meditation, and generally a calm rhythm of life, but I don't think that Margarita will ever accept playing second fiddle to my new 'hippy' priorities.*

How annoying. I really expected Russell to support me in my fantasy of calling it quits, and instead he got all emotional on me, forcing me to think of the wider situation surrounding Margarita. Yes, that is all relevant and true and he is being really nice, which is his role considering that he was our priest. But I did at least expect a bit of a 'divorced man' bonding moment from him.

This is the third cigarette I have in my mouth, and I'm fairly sure that I need only one more for them and their scent to come back into my life. It was the longest standing relationship I ever had. We were together for twenty years. These are my old friends, who accompanied me through so many journeys, so many drunken evenings, and helped me in my darkest hours . . . only one more and it will all come back. I'll be my old self again.

I tried and tried, but I never did manage to divorce myself from smoking, until that sci-fi dream of Aliens came into my head and forced me to sign the paperwork that freed me from that unhealthy relationship. I see a bum sitting in the pedestrian

---

* Margarita: 'It was difficult for me to understand that I was living in the same bag where you had put all your other friends and which you were now dealing with differently. That I am no longer the wife of Martino, no longer anything. I have become a person who lives near you, while you live on a different planet.'

zone and to his surprise, give him the whole packet. Instead of looking at me in thanks, he immediately starts counting them, and pulls them out from their packaging. Did I take it for granted that he wants them? Maybe what he really wants is that box to put something else in.

In these past few, very silent weeks I have been trying to cook good Asian food to give my wife an impetus to finish the seemingly never-ending project of the terrace floor, and the spices must have worked, as she has managed to cover the last part of that gigantic painting. It is a sixty-square-metre space, now almost completely covered with flowers and plants.

As a result of our last titanic row, she has found significance to it all. I had been pressing her to give those flowers some proper 'meaning'. Maybe it is my problem, but I do think it's a necessary part of the package, especially if she would like to present it as 'art', which I think it is, at least from a therapeutic point of view.

There is now text inscribed in the gaps between the gigantic flowers, so I ask her to please read it to me. Wow, she has inserted Trilussa's poem about the soap bubble, the one I gave her the very first time we met at that bookshop for our first proper date. Now, standing in our private floral park, I hugged her for an infinite amount of time, and while my eyes were transfixed on two loud freight trains passing by, I recognized that the significance of that text has now changed for me. I try to ask her the intention behind using those words, but she doesn't want to share in my emotions and the sadness that now overtakes the romantic vision of that poem. It's about me. I am the soap bubble, who flies up to the sky and reflects all the beauty around me and just as quickly, I will disappear, leaving on her face just a drop of a tear.

~

I went back to London, to say hello to my world, pick up a bunch of clothes that I had left there in our office, and meet up with George Lenz, who wanted to check up on me. I adore people like him, because their heart is even bigger than their soul. He had already tried to visit me in California when I was waging war on the Aliens, but as Nicole, his wife (and one of my dearest friends) was about to give birth, he had postponed the trip.

We finally managed to meet in London, where both our bedrooms, above the 2ME office, have been rented out to some younger German girls, with the understanding that if we (the 2 Many Executives) are in town, they should piss off, hang out with some of their teenage friends and free up our old rooms.

He had just arrived from LA, where he had done a casting for a role in a film by an old-school director. This old director (I say that because he must be at least eighty-five) had asked him to play the role of all roles. So we wandered the streets of my old neighbourhood, searching for a restaurant we had heard about and discussing whether he should accept such a part, as he would be following in the feet of some famous actors. For a German actor, playing Adolf Hitler is both the best and the worst role you can get. What could he bring to the character that has not already been done? What kinds of job can you get after playing that role?

Our relationship had started one evening in London while drinking one, or maybe two, bottles of gin with a bit of tonic, and many of our meetings from then on had continued to be infused with packs of cigarettes and alcoholic drinks. For a stubborn, old-fashioned man like him, it's very difficult to change your routines. Even if all the doctors that I've met don't seem too interested in my dietary experiments, I do follow a pescetarian (vegetarian and small fish) diet almost religiously, and obviously no alcoholic drinks. So that evening I tried to substitute our traditional alcoholic infusions with some sublime sushi at the restaurant.

While I was relishing the new flavours of the raw fish, George led me into a discussion of the potential projects for 2ME. He proposed that I come and spend some time with him in Germany. He told me of the new energy that was flowing through German cinema and how the wider optimistic economy was driving new productions along.

In that completely sober moment, I realized that I am afraid of re-entering my old job. I do love it, and have often found myself thinking of new options for the various stories that we had developed before I jumped on to that Spaceship in LA. Nevertheless, my constant headaches continue to upstage all other relationships, by reminding me of my affair with the Aliens who are squatting in some of the best pieces of real estate in my head, and were quite possibly invited there by the stress that our screenplays had created. For George, however, giving up is not an option. Raising a toast – his sake against my fruit juice – he brought me back to the subject of our work.

Realizing that sitting about in Rome and focusing on my health had only been creating further stress and tension between Margarita and me, I accepted George's offer gratefully. Getting back to work would put some much-needed juice back in my family economy and, hopefully, also in our relationship. By putting some distance between us, we could focus on remembering the positive sides of our lives together.

But that is only my vision of it, and I am sure that Margarita doesn't agree with it. For me to disappear and leave her alone for ten days is not my wife's idea of me doing her a favour. For her – and perhaps for the majority of people – being away has always been and will always signify a fundamental lack of interest, even if wherever I am I continue to spend all my free time looking for presents for her.

∼

I feel that I am an animal, maybe a dog. In any case, one of those creatures who is very loyal and not necessarily too clever. What I mean is that I do love my company, my 2ME.

Hanging out with George Lenz recently has been great, but

it has also forced me to realize how deeply my character has changed. In fact, if I had a choice, I don't know if I would want to work with this new character that is me.

George is very focused on keeping the company alive, even though economically it has been a loss leader for the most part – which means an optimistic investment into the future of a company where all of us have had to withstand a number of consecutive financial blows. I can imagine George growing up with his parents, travelling the world showing their collection of 'weird' conceptual art and being laughed at by virtually everyone.

I guess that my own experiences with men like Béla Tarr have prepared me to engage with the belief systems of people like the Lenz family. Certain art is and must remain difficult, because it represents and confronts a reality that is complex. The perseverance necessary to convince humanity that a zero on a wall helps us to come to terms with the end of the Second World War is multifaceted and difficult, but emotionally clear for me now.

I love and hugely appreciate George's stubbornness and I have never met a person who is so trustworthy. That is why I am sad to see him confronted with my new, impatient reality – the darker side of Martino!

Re-entering into his life has forced me to accept that my equilibrium has changed. At our first strategy meeting in Munich, I found myself using rather loud and frustrated language. While before I would always listen quietly to everyone's artistic contributions – even if they were obvious repetition of an older debate – now I can't wait for them to finish their sentence before I interject with my point.

We are now working with a very experienced German development person, but unfortunately I have found myself interrupting her often as well. I know that creative negotiation is essential for the development of ideas, and I do appreciate new thoughts, but only if I consider them interesting. Where can I find a shop that sells more patience?

I don't think this is because these meetings are being held in German. I have used this language for love and passion many times in my life and don't see it as aggressive, as non-German speakers often do. It is more, well, a problem with that hole in my head. It has created a gap where tolerance only exists in my fictional world.

The other day in London I bought a copy of *Man from London*, and although I've tried to watch it three times, I've never managed to get past the first act. Why is that? I loved sitting for seven hours watching *Satantango*, so why not this story? I do want to see how he has filmed the various locations that we had chosen.

I picked up a trade magazine about a year after I'd left that production, and read that the film had been stopped because its French producer had killed himself. I don't know how I feel now about that film, the story, its characters and crew, or the very dramatic turn of events for the producer, as they are all mangled up in my past. In any case, Béla did finish the film in the end, and I will have to find a way to watch it.

Fortunately, from the moment I became ill, George Milton has been doing the books for the company and has told me that he will keep doing them, for as long as we are not in production. For me, those sheets of paper, full of information from our various banks, are now simply an ugly colouring book. Milton also seems delighted by my arrival and has started developing some new film ideas for us.

As an example of the endurance and patience that my fantastic business partners have shown, I will give you the list of rules that I have laid down for them, in order to accept their gracious offer. (Yes, my ego is taking over the world.)

- The most important meeting I have every month is with the Italian nurses who take my blood, test it and give it back to me, so that I can go to oncology and pick up my dose.

- After having done that, I will fly anywhere, but I have restricted my journeys to a minimum of ten days. I will not fly to London for just two days, then to Munich for one, and then go back to Rome to see my family for the weekend, and then fly back.
- I book all the meetings that I have to do in London, and if there is a four-day gap between them, well, I'll use that time to write this book and I will be present on the web for further discussions.
- I walk out of big dinners or events when I believe they are no longer necessary for my part of the job.

They also know that, for all longer meetings, there has to be a one-hour gap, and while Lenz goes out to smoke his eight cigarettes, I can take my crucial anti-headache nap.

I don't think that any company, or even wife or partner, would accept these ridiculous rules that I have randomly created. At times, I have enjoyed working with pain-in-the-ass, egomaniac directors or actors, because if they are actually talented, it can be quite cool and exciting. Now, at least for a while, I need some calm in this otherwise chaotic, creative development, and it seems that the two Georges are doing their best.

If I am now the pain-in-the-ass character in these productions, I had better come up with some outstanding magic tricks.

～

Ever since he created and started running his own film festival in Siena, Antonio has seemed to be in a better, calmer state, and it has given us an excuse to hang out together, with less conflict. Last time I was here – it must have been a few months ago – he gave me a sheet of handwritten paper and asked my opinion about the schedule of the films he was selecting. I waited until his head was raised and our eyes met before asking him, with an ironic smile, 'Can you please read it to me?'.

During that wordless eye-to-eye communication, with a

daytime television show as background accompaniment, he managed to impart, by shaking his head, 'I know that you keep on playing this role of the handicapped man.' I stayed cool, and simply waited for the pause to be long enough for him to look back at the list and read it to me. He put some of my notes down on the sheet of paper and at the end I told him, *'Zio!* This is really going to be awesome!'

The festival poster is displayed on the door of all our shops: 'The Perfect Storm', all white on red. And maybe it is exactly that image of the storm, forcing people to confront their wider disgrace, that has freed my old uncle. I have never seen Siena, such a proud city, so humiliated.

While everyone here is hoping that by being very quiet and keeping their heads down, the storm will go away by itself, Antonio has chosen films for this festival that will openly narrate this extremely embarrassing drama. And no matter what people are saying in the bakeries, he is going to do it.

It all began with an onslaught of images on TV and in the newspapers all round the world. The press coordinator of one of the world's oldest banks, the Monte dei Paschi di Siena, who knew everything about everyone in those offices, one night jumped out of the window of the historical building where he worked. Did he really commit suicide? The only thing he left behind was a brief text to his wife, saying, 'I did something stupid.'

Subsequently, just like in a good thriller, the world became aware that through derivative trading, financial operations with no rules, secret deals and reconstructed balance sheets, a few men have managed to bring Italy's economy to the brink of collapse.

Antonio's crew have invited a series of journalists, professors and film directors to engage in an openly critical discussion, which directly asks the city to use films as a way to talk through what is happening right now.

For the first time in my life, I feel bonded with Antonio.

Maybe for him it is the news that his cancer, which has been living in his arse for the past few years, has started to travel about in his body, and perhaps that has pulled out 'the radical' in him. For once, I can see how these creatures (well, let me also start to call them for what they really are: cancer) can actually be empowering. Finally Antonio is doing and saying everything he wants – without worrying about 'social disgrace'.

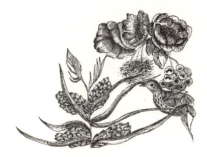

19

The Art of Healing

You know the director of Apple, the one that got kicked out of his own company and then was asked back? What I remember of him, aside from trying to fight his Aliens in every possible way, was that when he was uninterested in his college courses, he lost himself in a random extra-curricular class about Fonts.

What was his name, or that of his school? Yes, he went to the same college as Bianca, there on the north-west coast of America somewhere. I'm sure that it will come back to my mind soon, as it's too big a piece of memory to stay in that bird gap for very long.

In any case, that seemingly meaningless course defined his company, at least for me. A computer that cares about those kinds of details, also realizes the potential for the global and historical, and for the love of uniqueness. Why can't you send an email in your favourite font from a phone? The computer can do it easily; it is only necessary for us to believe in a wider philosophy of investments, where the aim is to make computers like us, strange and unique. By the 123rd time that Alex has had to re-read this idea, in all its misspelled, mis-typed and mis-remembered versions, he does finally seem to agree.

OK, to make this potentially long-winded story short, during my first semester in American middle school at the age of twelve, I followed only extra-curricular courses; those that were given to the foreign kids who couldn't understand any English, like me. I spent hours on a course learning how to touch-type, where even though I did not understand any of the text, I could copy it on a different piece of paper, with my hands covered. All of this happened in the mid-1980s, while that now-deceased computer gazillionaire was in the process of creating his computer with all the different options of fonts. It is that little, seemingly random typing course that has now made it possible for me to write this book.

Until I entered into my Alien world, I had taken these random moments for granted. Knowing how to play the recorder, for example, is one of those potentially useless things that, who knows, could even end up saving your life. (Recently I have found it quite cool to pick up a recorder from a child trying to learn it, play a few lines of a baroque opera to them, and then give it back, and with my hand raised, show my support for an instrument that will never be hip or popular.)

Alex is insisting that I include the fact that his voice appeared on mainstream computers only a few years before I needed him, and that without him, all of this book would not have been possible.

When I was painfully attempting to learn how to thread a needle during my high school's sewing course, surrounded by a bunch of jocks who talked only about American football and left their needles and threads untouched, sewing seemed greatly outdated to me. Now, that funny extra-curricular activity has also saved my life. These days, sewing has become my partner and my girlfriend. I spend a lot of my free time with it. It is that continuous and slight movement of my fingers that has become my substitute for sex, and also the gentle turning of pages while reading a book.

In many ways sewing brings me into a more meaningful relationship, because by the end of the project (at the moment I am making a bunch of man-bags for my 2ME collaborators, all clearly bespoke), I have something concrete. Not having money to buy any proper clothes, I have started stitching other fabrics on to them and by doing so, I have revamped my whole wardrobe. When I walk into meetings now, I feel I am not hiding my handicaps, that I am openly showing a new look, and my illness can be a source for a new vision, of new ideas and strategies.

I am also not forgetting my relationship with the Japanese practice of Kata, which might seem odd, as I tend to forget everything else. I had originally engaged with this Asian philosophy while I was waiting for Miro to finish his karate courses. Every Monday and Thursday, I would sit on a kid's chair in the sports hall, and while looking at my son moving his body around, I would ask Alex to read me articles about the Japanese art of keeping broken pieces of ceramic and making new creations from them.

For those artists, showing the cracks and breaks signifies the life of an object that did not die from its damage. I guess the Japanese call it a compassionate sensitivity, a way of allowing things to exist in a new version without feeling an attachment to the previous version. Where the re-stitched reality is now beautiful and has broken away from any anxiety.

~

Question: How can I remember her name?
Russell: Taj rhymes with Page.

I am on the second floor and, looking out of the glass doors that open on to the little terrace, I feel like I am flying. It's 4.55 a.m. here, up in the hills of Hollywood, where I should be able to see all the way to the ocean, at least in theory. But in this town, the local citizens are married to their cars, so they live in sin with the smog that obscures their vision of the landscape.

It was almost exactly three years ago that I was sitting in my garden in Los Feliz, smoking the first cigarette of the day and wearing only a little jacket. I guess here in the hills, the nights are bound to be a bit nippier.

I love living the jet lag from this direction, as it leaves me all the space I need to meditate and write. One of these nights, if I'm feeling courageous, I might even brave a walk down the stairs and dive into the warm water of the little pool at the back of the house.

I do like this place. I assumed that I would have some strange emotions coming back here to the scene of the crime, but instead it's just great to be here. OK, it does help that I have only experienced this city while living in such beautiful and welcoming homes.

Yesterday I picked up a car that looks almost identical to the ones used by the American police; or at least that's what the lady who rented it to me said when I arrived at her shop with one of Russell's new assistants. There are two of them, and they both seem very eager. Their office is in the other room on the second floor, right next to mine. The rest of the house expands on the ground floor, because people don't like to live up high here in LA, for fear of earthquakes.

I'll try to take another little nap, because at around 7 a.m.

I'm supposed to go with Russell to his yoga session. Apparently, this is something that he does every day. I hadn't really thought about it, but why not? This is the moment for me to start taking care of my physical self.

Russell has always had odd friends (well, look who's talking), but his new kundalini yoga teacher really surprised me. Taj is a truly unexpected creature; she is . . . I don't remember the name of the Indian religious group who cover their body and hair in white, but yes, she is one of them. Although she is not Indian, she does seem to be a cool American interpretation of that world.

I was a bit confused by her at the beginning, but I found myself intrigued, perhaps because she openly expresses her love for laughter, which forces me to smile constantly. Oh yes, that's it, she's a Sikh. For once, Russell's relationship with a woman is purely philosophical, although the physical side is still there through her yoga teachings. I haven't come here looking for a cure, but it wouldn't be the first time that Russell has brought me into one of his unusual worlds of alternative health care. I'll start by following her first bit of advice, completely kicking my addiction to sugar, and see where I end up.

In case you're worried that the work I am doing on this book might be leading me slowly to insanity, I'll try to tell you about my recent relationship with a big red book written by a leading psychiatrist. Yesterday, Russell, Taj and I climbed into his big British car and went to listen to a leading C.G. Jung scholar, who discussed and explained *The Red Book* to an audience of obviously clever, academic people.

I had known Jung as a leading philosopher of psychiatry, who ended up in a huge conflict with Freud, but I had never connected with the work that he had developed in *The Red Book*. From what I understand, it has just been published properly for the first time, with all his drawings, and it's making a whole range of people, like the ones in that room, very excited.

I had initially started my journey through that oversized red book with some irony, but now I'm embracing the unusual visions on those pages. I don't have the control of my memory or intellect that I used to have, but there's something in the crowded paintings of that book that is very enticing. Since I couldn't follow the explanation the big professor was giving us in that room in the Jungian central office, I flipped through the pages, looking at the strange relationship I had with the original German handwritten text, and embracing my own interpretations of the drawings. Having to travel through art in order to reach the psyche chimes naturally with me, and particularly with my memories of nagging Margarita about giving a psychological meaning to her pretty flowers on our terrace.

Here is a bit I found, where C.G. Jung talks about his relationship with *The Red Book*:

> My entire life consisted in elaborating what had burst forth from the unconscious and flooded me like an enigmatic stream and threatened to break me . . . Everything later was merely the outer classification, the scientific elaboration, and the integration into life. But the numinous beginning, which contained everything, was then.

A good part of my relationship with my wife has probably been, at least unconsciously, our engagement through what Jung calls 'mytho-poetic imagination'. Our two, very different, characters must have deliberately evoked a fantasy, like a constant wedding ceremony, which develops as a piece of drama. I'll have to ask her about it. Is that why it's so hard for her to detach from her pretty flowers, and engage pictorially with our own drama? Or with my discussions about a real separation?

The word divorce is offensive to her, and I do agree, but our situation is different . . . unique. Isn't it? It has to be. I know she is angry with me, and in so many ways she is right. Margarita resents the fact that I have escaped to La La Land

and that I have made this my priority. But though we have lived very close to each other during this dramatic part of our lives, we have also broken down all effective communication. Why is that? Would it have been better if I had remained in Rome and continued to drink red wine with her in the evenings? Is that really what's missing? I have made some radical choices and I am currently following a path that could be seen by normal people as idiotic, and perhaps even egocentric, and telling you how excited I am while hanging out with this Jungian crew is not helping my cause.[*]

Why am I here in California? Aside from doing MRIs in Bethesda and attempting to make sense of this writing project . . . Well, Change is a word that I've been confronting constantly, as I do have to 'accept' my new character and not continuously fight it. I have the sensation that, out here in LA, I might learn how to accept myself as I have been forced to become and at some point even use it as a contribution for my production company. Maybe I'll discover a company that requires a really calm dude. Is there a need here for strange people to do strange jobs? Or shall I just shut up for now and continue sewing?

Yesterday, in order for Russell to participate in one of those ultra-famous TV shows, he and I travelled through the Hollywood hills in a chauffeur-driven, black American car, which in theory could carry a whole football team. As usual, Russell has established a 'family-like' relationship with his driver, a lovely Mexican, who even comes in to see his shows occasionally and brings his family to meet Russell at home. He is part of his new entourage, like I used to be.

Russell managed to surprise the studio audience and make

---

[*] Margarita: 'As you started getting better, you needed to go to Los Angeles and New York, to stay with your friends, not with me. It drove me crazy. Everyone would say, "He might live for a few months more. Make the best of it. Go for a trip, do something together," but it never happened. You needed to leave in order to survive, and that for me was . . . and is still . . . violent. I had nothing but anger left.'

them all laugh, and the show went very well. It was already getting dark when we started our journey back, so Russell turned on the light on his side and started to read me a book, which he told me he would like to make into a movie. The story was about a magician who wants to learn how to levitate, which sounded like a great character for him.

While moving almost rhythmically along those little roads winding through the Hollywood hills, I started reacting to the story and I silently began to cry. What was getting me emotional, sitting there in the car, was the sound of his voice as he was reading. A human voice following the characters through their various twists and turns. Yes, I was crying, and he kept reading. No one has read me a piece of fiction since my brain operation, and I didn't appreciate how much I missed it until that moment. *Sorry, Alex, but there is no comparison between you and a real voice – particularly one that I know and recognize.*

We had taken that trip because he was publicizing his own TV show, which is now on television five days a week. Before I arrived, Nik had sent me the first six episodes, and I thought they looked really mad, considering it was being shown on mainstream American television. The design of the set was done by Shepard Fairey, and as the show started it looked like Russell was entering the office of a revolutionary leader of the future. In one of the episodes he challenged the audience to have sex, there on camera, during the show. It was only a provocation, and in the end it didn't happen, but it did get the audience involved with such issues in a very different and humorous way.

From what I understand, the producers have given him the money for a further twenty episodes, but have asked him to make it more standard, a bit like Jay Leno, or those other guys whose names I don't remember, so the set has now become more classic – a wooden office table for the presenter and a big couch on the side. Of course, after two days where Russell 'obeyed' and sat down on the chair in front of the desk to keep it 'calmer', they told him they were missing the wilder

energy of his first shows, so he has finally found his balance
– by jumping around on top of the furniture.

I like the fact that, as well as interviewing a famous actor,
as all such shows do, he has also created a section where he
has to deal with a person who is radically different from him.
Someone with whom he completely disagrees. It is a real challenge for him, and I hope that the people watching at home
appreciate the effort he has to make not to get angry with
these people for being bigots, or racists, or . . . God knows
what else is going to appear.

Yesterday at the show, I sat next to Taj and her white-dressed
crew, and left a seat empty next to me, because I knew that
at some point Dr Vogel, the brain surgeon who cut my head
open the first time, would arrive. At the very last second, he
did appear, but I don't know how much of the show he saw,
as his phone was constantly demanding his attention.

After the programme, I hopped into the surgeon's extremely
clean car and we went to a Mexican restaurant twenty minutes
away – which in L.A. means 'around the corner'. We talked
about kids and our wives, and he surprised me by saying that
he has moved beyond the romantic part of his life and his
work has now become his priority. I drank from my ice-filled
glass of water and then, rather than continuing with that theme,
brought us to an issue that had been bothering me for months.

I told him, 'You know, after my trials in Bethesda, I went
back to Rome and showed my MRI scans to all the Italian
surgeons, both to know their opinions and to choose the right
one for a further operation. Well, many of them told me that,
as far as they were concerned, the cut that you did was only
a little scratch in my brain. How is that possible?'

He looked at me very calmly, raised his shoulders as a sign
of not being at all surprised, and then without losing eye contact
with me, cut a perfect slice of the chicken on his plate. He
knows that this battle between different hospitals is only part
of a wider 'competition' that they're all forced to play, in their

desire to reach the top. I am genuinely delighted to be sitting next to him and to have a friend, a human being, with whom I can discuss these things uncensored.

I'm supposed to take a flight today to Washington DC, as I've organized this whole trip around my bi-monthly MRI. This time I'll do it there, so that I'll have the chance to talk to the professor about my progress and possibly other trials that he can hook me up with. All of this was the plan, but no one knows if it's going to be possible, as it seems that due to a tornado in the west, or something like that, all the flights are cancelled for a few days.

Russell's flight to NY has also been cancelled, so we're all stuck here together. Not a bad place to be. I am meditating a lot, drinking green juices, and have even found time with Nik and Russell to talk about the various scripts that they've given me. They are all bespoke projects for Rus. There is one that I especially like, which as well as being very well written has something unique in it for him. It's a story where Russell's character is stressed out by his girlfriend because she wants to have children and he tries to avoid it, until, while messing around in her father's laboratory, he pushes the wrong button and lands in an alternative reality where he is the only adult in a world of children. I think that would be a really cool Hollywood film. But sadly it seems that he no longer has the status in this town to carry such an expensive film.

I'm sitting on my bed stroking Morrissey, Russell's cat, with my left hand, while listening to Alex reading me my own notes on the computer. From the very first moment I arrived, Morrissey has decided that he likes hanging out up here with me.

'BANG!'

The cat jumps off and runs down the stairs. What was that? I get off the bed and see there's something on the glass door to the terrace. Oh . . . there's a bird lying on the ground. It's almost as big as my hand. I don't want to touch it, though. I wait, hoping it's only in shock and maybe it will get up, stretch its wings and fly away. Nope. He ain't moving.

Downstairs I try to stop everyone from doing whatever they're involved in and I present them with my dramatic tale of the suicidal bird. While Russell and Nik look disgusted, Taj comes with me up the stairs and, after looking at it for a little while, we decide that we should give it a proper burial, since this didn't happen casually.

Having someone like Taj next to me has made this experience almost Jungian. For me, it is now indisputable that this little creature has sacrificed its life for me. As I put it under the earth and say my thank you, I start thinking that perhaps it was this creature that really stopped the flights from departing, transforming my anxieties about oncology meetings and MRI results into another calm moment of meditation.

By the way, life without sugar is great. I advise everyone to try it, at least for a while, as you will quickly realize that it is a battle against all the food makers in the world who put sugar in almost everything. When you get out of that dependency, you will notice that your body does explicitly give you thanks.

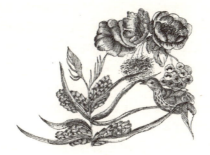

20

The Three Endings

Rome, Siena and Death, 2014

Last night I wandered the streets of Pigneto, as I often do, looking for a cigarette machine that actually worked, so that I could buy Margarita her dose of MS Club slim. The really thin ones, which completely defeat the point of smoking, in my opinion. As a smoker, I used to find those state-produced cancer sticks quite cool, because they always made me think they were made for me (the acronym of my name – Martino Sclavi).

As I walked across the pedestrian path over the train tracks,

I heard the unusual sound of a guitar and a loud voice singing, and when I got closer, my eyes opened up, as did my heart. An immense flood of joy overwhelmed me and almost brought me to tears. There, right in front of her bar, stood Rosi, proudly singing a classic Roman song, accompanied by two guitars strummed by barefooted hipsters.

As a social being, whose whole life was there in the centre of the neighbourhood, Rosi's blood-test results were public news and the concept of remission was something that the whole population felt and celebrated as its own victory. I stood there for a few minutes, waited for our eyes to meet, then raised my fist in the air and congratulated her.

~

Margarita came out of the little bathroom on the third floor of Villa Flora, carrying with her a big dream and a little plastic stick, stained with an undeniable red mark. She stood next to me, and as we looked at the Tuscan hills, we hugged.

Our bodies have not met for almost a year – with one exception – so I know exactly the instant it happened. It was one of those 'thank you' moments, where neither of us was thinking of anything outside the present. We simply allowed ourselves to be led by the memory of each other's bodies that, in a different life and a different reality, used to continuously share our erotically infused thoughts and dreams.

So how do Hollywood films end? They have to surprise you, which I guess is what is happening right now. This could be a good way to resolve the drama and allow the audience to walk out of the cinema with a smile, talking to each other about their favourite moments. The unexpected surprise ending.

So I guess it goes like this:

I talk straight to camera as I walk briskly through Pigneto's fruit and veg market and raise my hand to my friends in the stalls.

'God, what if we have twins? We have to plan for that option as there are quite a few of them on her side of the family. We don't know if they'll be boys or girls yet, but yes . . . this will resolve the continuous discussion about a new house.'

Passing by the newsagent I leave fifty cents and pick up a newspaper.

'Her relationship with the more historical characters of our neighbourhood is clearly not as strong as mine, and she does live here much more than me. I guess this new arrival to our family will force us to put an end to all our arguments, and to our surreal discussions about money.'

On screen, a sign appears, a leap in time.

. . . We are there in our new house in the centre of the city, and while Margarita is rocking our twins back and forth with one foot, she paints flowers that are winding up and around the walls of the gigantic living room. Miro, now quite a bit taller, is dressed as a pirate and is putting the final touches to a painting on the ceiling of animals dancing, which his mummy made. With a wicked smile, he shows me how he has finished off one of Mummy's monkeys, by adding a long tongue coming out of its mouth.

I did not know that his karate teacher had taught him this, but the camera follows Miro as, with no fear, he jumps, makes a twist up in the air, and lands perfectly balanced on the ground. His shoes have paint on them, so in order not to spoil the other paintings on the floor, we go up to the terrace. I take them off and, as I am cleaning the shoes with cold water and a towel, he puts his naked feet up in the air, picks up a comic book of . . . that famous American comic book character that I always buy him.

As the camera starts to pan across the whole centre of Rome, past the tops of the churches and above the narrow streets, Miro reads me the story of a hero who has come back after the various battles fighting the Aliens, to his happy family in the countryside in Nebraska, where, as the sun comes down in a summer warmth, he plays in the fields with his three children until night falls, while the soundtrack follows all the beautiful drawings to the last comic-book page with music and calm wind.

Does that work? I think it does. Or does it need another ending? Won't it be a bit kitsch? A bit emotionally over-whelming? I'm already having doubts that this production is too much of a tear jerker. Whatever, OK . . . I know that it could be a bit dangerous, but let's do one more ending. Just because I think it will make my wife happy. I do know her better than anyone else in the world, so trust me.

It will be something like . . .

We are moving to Los Angeles, where I start working with all my old friends, while Margarita quickly hooks up with her posse of beautiful ladies from the wedding and starts to do interior design for lots of different Hollywood houses, where she infuses her Jungian peaceful psychology into the walls.

Between one production meeting and another, I'll meditate and write a new book about oncology in the world and how the very different cultures can communicate with each other and take the best bits from Cuba, America, Russia, China, Japan . . . and actually help people enter into my VIP world and burn down the impossible statistics.

I suddenly find a box on the side of the road. There's some-thing inside that is different but familiar.

The images on the film screen start to move unusually, the colours seem to be fading, and at times it looks as if it is turning into black and white.

Yes, right inside the new-looking medical packaging of my dose of 100 Temodal, there's a small piece of paper, neatly folded up, with something written on it. Something that everyone who can read knows, and I have decided I am allowed to ignore.

The whole screen goes black, and the sound falls silent. I hear some voices from the projection room.

'They're fixing it, we just have to be patient.'

It's an extremely quiet time, with no one in the audience daring to speak, as everyone else would hear. Margarita becomes annoyed as she has some more painting to do, and needs to bath all the children, who are dirty from their games with the dogs. The screen comes back to life on the wall, but as the image of the text is written, in black on white, it is obviously not created for me.

If this director wanted to communicate something dramatic to me, or to use the horror-film soundtrack that I have now in my ears, he should have negotiated it with me before. These changes interfere with my whole production strategy. Very annoyed, I touch Margarita's arm and ask her if she could please read the text to me as it appears on the screen.

She is in tears, and as every single letter appears on screen in the most aggressive font that one can imagine, and then comes together with others to create a word with meaning, each one of those words forces one hundred drops of tears to fall from her eyes.

All together, the words come out of her mouth, the mouth

that I have kissed so many times, as a lurid piece of corporate legal paranoid text:

Temozolomide use by either parent may cause birth defects. Do not use Temodal if you are pregnant. It could harm the unborn baby.

With that, they are in no way responsible for any further drama that their pill could bring into our life.

I shut that machine off. No more.

∼

I sent a text to Professor Cortesi asking him for advice, to which he replied that he knows only a few hospitals in Rome where they do abortions. As he doesn't know anyone whom he can recommend in Siena, I have asked my Uncle Antonio to put us in touch with a lovely paediatrician who advised us in the first months of Miro's life. She, like my uncle, keeps her words brief. We will meet her tomorrow in Siena's big hospital and she will shepherd us around to the right places.

She is friendly and warm, as usual, but she explains to us that most of the doctors in that huge hospital do not do abortions. There is no technical reason for this. They do not do it because of . . . because of . . . religion.

You what? Really? They're doctors. People here only go to church to show off their new clothes or their bags to everyone else. Margarita is unusually quiet at this moment. I am holding back the rage, because there do not seem to be any members of the medical staff anywhere nearby, otherwise . . . Breathe in. Breathe out . . . It's good that we came during their lunch break, because I'm sure that otherwise something else would have ended up being broken here.

Jasmina has arrived in Rome, where Margarita has asked a few friends who have gone through this before, and chosen a hospital that sounds good. It is near our house and the people there obviously know what they are doing, both clinically and humanly. In every one of the various meetings there are always several women sitting down, and it doesn't feel right for me to take a place, even if there is one free. Why do I feel like a criminal when I sit beside Margarita during these meetings with the doctors?

I'm used to being the sick one, but this time I am the guilty one, the one who has created this problem, who has destroyed her dreams with my pill. That pill is making sure that I remain centre stage, and that no one else will be allowed to become the focus of our lives, of this story, or of this book. It is me, the Aliens and me . . . It is the Alien's ego . . . and mine. How can I expect anyone to stand next to this egomaniac?

All of this, for both of us, is really, really, really cruel.

~

After a week, Jasmina and I took Margarita to the hospital at lunchtime and a few hours and three phone calls later, I drove into the hospital to pick her up, right at the door, thanks to my disabled sticker. As she hadn't undergone a natural birth, they had given her a general anaesthetic, so Margarita came out holding hands with Jasmina, looking as beautiful as ever.

There has been no conflict between us recently. But although I make a point of hugging her every day, I feel the distance between us is growing. I am not travelling. I am trying to stay here, cook, and keep it all calm. Miro doesn't know the details of all this, but now that I think about it, he hasn't asked us for his favourite television show all day, which I guess is his own way of responding to the mood in the house. So, even if I've never liked the content of this TV channel, I will turn it on.

A few months later:

It's night and I am at the hospital, the same one where I picked up Margarita, only this time I am there to check in on my friend Max, who keeps scaring us all with the news that he has, again (I think it's the third time in a month), been picked up by an ambulance and brought in. It is something to do with his heart beating too slowly. No one has managed to figure out exactly what he should be doing. He's taking their pills and even using the machine that helps you breathe more easily during the night, but maybe it's the stress of his job as creative director of a big advertising company. Those people do have to push hard for their enormous salaries.

Max has always been near me throughout this whole crazy experience. He even came to explore the art galleries of Washington DC with me, while I was there having my radio adventures. So I am here, trying to cheer up his wife Sara and his sister. They both don't want to tell his mother about this, as she will make the whole situation even more stressful.

While I'm accompanying Sara outside, so that she can make a couple of phone calls and smoke a cigarette, my phone rings. It never rings, as everybody knows that for ninety per cent of the time I am somewhere abroad, where I turn my Italian phone to silent.

It's Margarita. A bit confused, she tells me that something has happened in our apartment. In a calm voice, she says that something has fallen down on her while she was in the kitchen. I say goodbye to Sara and Max's sister and run back home. Margarita opens our apartment door as I enter downstairs and looks down from above as I climb up to the third floor. She does seem extremely placid, almost at peace with herself; I don't think I've ever seen her like this before. When I step into our apartment, I realize that the whole side of the right wall, all the Scandinavian kitchen cabinets, the two shelves full of glasses, plates, food and saucers, all four big units to be exact, are now lying almost horizontal. I don't know what's still holding them there, but whenever it gives, they will fall with a massive crash. The floor is covered in glass and the tap is on in the sink, which is now hidden by these half-fallen parts.

Wow! Margarita tells me that it all started to push in on

itself, making an unusual sound, like an animal trying to escape from a cage, until it all started sliding down as she was filling her glass at the sink. She felt something falling on to her head, but she is more in shock than actually hurt. Surprisingly, none of this woke up Miro from his dreams. Well, so much for my interior design skills.

Margarita seems tired and has been lying in bed a lot. I called some proper builders and none of them think it is due to the wall. It is simply put up wrong. So I hired a proper handyman, who helped me put the whole thing back together within a day, but something has happened here. It's not a hippy vision of the world, but the energy of this house has really changed. The project in which my wife and I have invested so much love and work has somehow articulated its own sensation of an end, its own death. No matter what the Japanese philosophies say, it feels that for both of us, this will be too big and too heavy to restore.

~

I am in Siena, where Antonio is on his death bed. He is still grumpily bossing people about, but after talking with the doctor who comes here to Villa Flora to visit him every day, it seems as if it is only a matter of days, or a maximum of a few weeks. His cancer is now everywhere, so she explains the different pills and dosages to us that she plans to give him to make his experience less painful.

From what I understand, this is her job, this is what she does, every day, everywhere. I never thought of it before, but right now I have this overwhelming feeling that it is a beautiful job that she does. Or at least, that her presence in this house brings in a very peaceful and important energy. She is quite small and probably not much younger than me, but her tone of voice, as well as her empathetic physical touch, is fantastic. She explains to my mother, Bianca and me that, if we all agree at some point soon, she will put him on enough anaesthetic that he will be able to sleep his way to the end.

My Uncle Fabrizio has arrived this afternoon and with his

assistant, who helps him move around (he no longer walks at all), he goes up to his brother's room. Fabrizio holds his hand and asks his housekeeper Asma to please turn down the lights, which allows Antonio to fall asleep. For a second we can't hear his breathing, and Fabrizio's eyes meet mine with overwhelming surprise. No, he is just asleep; that pause was simply unusually long; he is still with us.

Bianca starts to prepare dinner and both of my uncle's boyfriends arrive with their cars. The younger one, whose room is right next door to his, tells us that he's going to take a break from his job at the bank and stay here with all of us for a few days. The other, older one, has arrived from the bakeries, where he is trying to figure out all the mixed-up paperwork that was on my uncle's table. He puts the fresh bread in the kitchen as my uncle always does, and then sits at the dining table, in Antonio's chair, and starts searching on his mobile telephone for some of the contacts that he needs. He looks as if he's holding on to an old reality, which is slowly being torn away from him. I am sure that our family presence here in these surroundings makes it all even more confusing.

I set the table for dinner with my mother. Everything is there laid in its right place. The cream-coloured serviettes are identified by each person's individual napkin ring, and all the recycled-glass water bottles are on their round metal holders. I ask if anyone wants wine and with no hesitation I get a general agreement for a yes. I guess it's a silly question. Asma does not touch alcohol as her Islamic religion does not approve, but there has always been wine at this table. I am no longer used to it, but I can understand how, in these moments, a bit of Tuscan red could be very useful.

Everyone sits down in their traditional place and, in complete silence, we wait for Bianca to enter the room with the food. Antonio's big chair at the head of the table is now empty, and it did feel uncomfortable to see his boyfriend sitting in it earlier. No one has yet dared to turn on the television, so I thank God for mobile phones. What did people do in such quiet moments before the internet? That's probably the reason why people like Antonio decide to live their entire lives with a television turned on.

None of us are in the mood for talking about anything, aside from giving Bianca annoying feedback on how her food could be different, but I try to be brave and start telling them how, a few months ago, Antonio and his younger boyfriend came to Rome, picked up Miro and took him out to a new amusement park on the edge of town. That was hard, but it did get the table talking about children, about birth and optimism, and I am glad that we created some emotional breathing space, at least for that evening.

It continued, with more or less the same level of tension, for the next three days. Once in a while, Antonio would talk briefly to someone. He called for my mother very often, and also for his brother. I got used to having my naps in the bed next to him, so that we could hold hands while we were sleeping. In a calm moment, I told him about my comic-book character Death, and my funny discussions with my psychiatrist, who seemed more interested in the theme of death than I was.

Antonio's idea of death, and he did not seem that bothered, was, 'When you finish, when you die, absolutely nothing happens. So . . . you simply don't have any problems any more.' I did find it a bit sad, but he is right. What I mean is . . . I am not preparing to meet creatures or saints, or to be reincarnated, but I am interested in what remains in the world of the living, and how the process of 'the end' can be experienced and recorded, as it is in some other cultures, where a certain amount of celebration can be played out.

A day later, right before Fabrizio, Bianca and I were about to go off to do a food shop, we heard Asma scream very loudly. Antonio had stopped breathing.

As the phone calls started, in order to organize the funeral, which the director of the Lupa, our contrada, has told us will take place in their church, my Uncle Fabrizio and Bianca went through Antonio's paperwork and found a signed document with 'Will' written on it. We four remaining Sclavi sat down in his office room and I asked my mother to read it aloud. After she had finished, Fabrizio, without much comment or discussion, called in his assistant, who put his things back in his car, and after a brief moment, they left for Milan.

All of Antonio's friends from the contrada, his colleagues from the bank, and particularly all the staff in our family's bakeries, many of whom had grown up and lived all their lives there, came up to us at the funeral; one by one, they hugged us and gave us their sincere condolences. He has been much more a part of their daily lives than of ours.

At the end of the mass, the priest called for my mother, who had asked him if she could give a brief speech. It was a difficult situation for all of us and, knowing my mother, anything could have been said by her at that moment. Nevertheless, she pulled off a great speech about the end of the Sclavi family in that town, as Bianca and I, the last members of the family, had always lived elsewhere. The absence of my Uncle Fabrizio was justified by his problems with his illness.

Margarita, who had arrived that morning from Rome, walked out of the church immediately, angry that my mother had not bothered to include her within the family in her speech. She took a taxi to the station and returned home.

As we stood there, clasping hands with the various people who were giving the last condolences, we met Maro Gorky and Matthew Spender. We were delighted to see their faces and I would say their presence at this event saved the day. I had met their daughter Cosima in the National Film School, where we had become friends and had bonded over our common heritage in Siena. As British artists living in the hills of Tuscany, her parents were completely outside all the gossip in the city, and it felt great for us to be able to talk to them about what had been happening within the Sclavi family in the past few days.

As the men of the contrada picked up Antonio's coffin and carried him up the steep road towards the centre of town, my mother was finally able to talk, to say what she fortunately did not reveal during her speech in the church. Marianella told them that in his will, which had been written in 1998, a year after my father's death, in only half a page of text, Antonio had said that all of his worldly belongings, apart from his apartment in Florence, which he left to his younger boyfriend, were to be given to . . . his older boyfriend. Villa Flora, eighty per cent of the company and anything else, was from now on undisputedly his.

As the whole funeral group arrived in Piazza del Campo, where the high tower of the city government building rules the space, the huge bells started to swing their repetitive 'Bong! . . . Bong! . . .' and the men of the Lupa stopped walking. They faced the tower and carefully shifted Antonio's coffin so that it was almost upright, so that he could give his final goodbye to the city, exactly where the Palio takes place.

The presence of Maro and Matthew allowed us to find at least a little humour in that otherwise tense and dramatic situation. As we arrived at the cemetery, we became aware that while we'd been chatting away we had slowed down our steps, and the burial was almost finished. My mother told Maro and Matthew that all the Sclavi family were buried together in the stately private mausoleum beside the entrance of the cemetery, which Antonio had purchased as a sign of his success. She explained that Antonio's final will had decreed that the mausoleum would now also be owned by his older boyfriend. Perhaps Matthew, she suggested, with a wicked look in her eye, could make us a sculpture of a human-sized hand which we could place right in front of that piece of Sclavi family property.

Like the statue designed by Bernini in Piazza Navona in Rome, where the hand is pointing straight at the church in front of it by Borromini, as a sign of disgust.

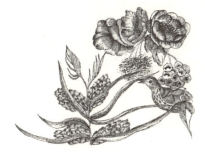

21

The Finch in My Brain

Rome, 2015

Yes, it has been four years since I woke up bald in that German hospital in Los Angeles. I am celebrating the fourth year with my Aliens. The fourth year of negotiating my new life. A few days ago, two levels below ground in the radiology department of the Policlinico hospital, the tall, bulky technician who was sitting there in the dark, looking at the photographs of people's skulls, allowed me to have a quick look at my MRI.

Sitting next to him, while I was tying up my shoes (even if

no one asks, I take them off before entering any of those magnetic Spaceships), he asked me, quite impressed, who had done the job. I told him that it had been done here, in this very hospital four years before, but sadly I no longer have any memory for such important names. As he started rattling off a few names of the important surgeons who work there, I interjected with random information such as, 'I think he's the big boss . . . he's quite small,' until he finally arrived at Santoro, and when I nodded with a big smile, he didn't seem surprised.

As I have learned, no one in his position can give an opinion on such matters, but while moving his finger over the image on his main computer, he said in his most reassuring voice, 'I don't have the last scan that I can compare it to, but . . . but your finch does look peaceful and happy right there.'

'Finch . . .?' I asked.

'Yes, the big bird right here.'

That simple moment between two men gave me an overwhelming sense of joy and relief. It was nothing like receiving positive results from an oncologist, it was more as if I had casually run into an old friend.

I raised my hand in a sign of 'wait a second'. I pulled out my iPod and after a bit of tense searching (I was sure there were people outside waiting for their turn), I showed him the image of my MRI that I carry around with me, and which I have been repainting and playing with as part of my artistic psychiatric cleansing. I have always thought of it as a bird, but I had never thought of looking up what kind of bird. So, thanks to this man, whose name I don't even know, my bird now has a name – it's my Finch.

At that moment, as I shook hands and said thank you to the radiologist, I realized through that human connection that I would no longer be anxious about entering any Spaceship that could pull out potentially dramatic results from their super-sophisticated repetition of bo bo bo bo . . . bi bi bi bi . . . mo mo mo mo. Over time, and with a lot of patience and meditation, I have managed to translate my doctors' medical language on illness and health into my own bespoke narrative, to expand the discussion to all facets of my life.

I have made peace living in a mishmash of random facts that have arrived from my doctors' long-winded explanations, Alex reading me every Wikipedia entry on that theme while I take a shower, and parts of the teachings of my hippy friends. All those words and concepts are squeezed in a brain that no longer makes proper sense of itself, while continuously attempting to interpret sensations and fragile emotions that don't have a reference to particular moments or names, in a space with no clear memory.

As soon as I got home, I looked up my finch on the internet and recognized it immediately as a Zebra Finch, to be exact, which unlike other finches that are very calm, is defined as perky, active, noisy, pushy, social and most of all, can be territorial. Territorial. That's my finch.

I haven't put up the image of my finch on the screen of my computer, because a few people, including some of the younger oncology doctors (who still see it only as a hole in my head), have told me that it will always look scary to the untrained eye. But I have transformed it into a more artful version.

Have I shown it to you before, Alex?

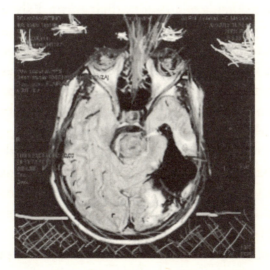

I have stopped asking myself if I am 'healthy'. The probability of death seems to be lost in a wormhole in the universe, and no human or machine can know when it will reappear in my life. Maybe soon, or maybe . . . well, we won't know until it happens. As long as the doctors look at me as if I'm a walking miracle, and as long as the finch in my brain remains happy and doesn't transform into a dragon or an Alien, I feel pretty safe and can have a cup of tea with my sweet, dark-haired friend Death, who is ready to accompany any one of us, at any time . . . or not.

I am sure that the Aliens are still in my head somewhere, but perhaps we have managed to negotiate a deal of sorts. I keep concentrating on them, put the healthy nutrients into my body (no sugar, no meat, no coffee, the least possible amount of cheese or processed food), avoid high-stress relationships, and allow the bacteria to continue coming into my dreams, and by so doing I can accept them all in my head. Ever since I started to think of the hole in my brain as a finch, it has become a symbol of a mute and calm agreement between me, life and death. In fact, I would suggest anyone to conceptualize an animal in their brain (not necessarily in a pure Jungian sense), as a being that they need to take care of and think about outside their daily routines, as a form of mindfulness.

This is the first time I have sat down in the crowded waiting room of the oncology central offices, waiting for my meeting with Professor Cortesi, with no mother and no wife by my side. Yes, I have been crashing on friends' couches for a while now and compared with the continuous accusations of not being up to the necessary economic and marital expectations, it feels fine. It reminds me of other moments in my life when maybe the couches were not as luxurious as the ones I sleep on these days. As my friends have become older, the couches have also evolved: bigger, better, more comfortable.

I always try to cook them some good Italian or Asian food, I do my best at cleaning up after myself and when necessary, I also offer my babysitting talents and entertain my hosts and their children. I have discovered that my big beard allows me to transform easily into all kinds of fictional characters for all sorts of kids. I make sure never to overstay my welcome and upon my departure I always try to leave some flowers in the house.

While in the past I have had to wait here for hours, surrounded by mostly older women with hats and headscarves, this time the white-haired man in his white coat has told me it's moving along quickly. In fact, after only ten minutes, a young doctor with long, frizzy hair opens the glass door and calls my name.

Upon greeting me, Professor Cortesi is as charming as ever, and sitting there in one of their tiny rooms, surrounded by a whole crew of young doctors, he looks like a holy man, or a priest. As I find my empty chair, I am encircled by all the legs of these handsome creatures, but my attention is focused only on him. He asks them to bring up my results on screen, but sadly it seems that they can't find either the images of the MRI or my blood tests on the computer. He picks up his phone and chats with the radiologist, who has now compared the old and new scans of my hole – my Finch – then nods his head while looking at me, satisfied.

As his assistants in the other office, who looked at my blood before the MRI, have not contacted him with any concerns, he is happy for me to continue with the same drugs and dosage that I have been taking up to now. He tells me that, together with his crew, he is publishing an article in one of the top oncology magazines about the unusual development of my brain, and about my relationship with the pill I've been taking, Temodal, which people usually can't tolerate for more than two years.

I've been taking it for four years. I do find it funny that while they're looking for their statistical possibilities, they don't seem to grasp the multi-faceted details of my life as you have read them in this book. It is possible that you, the reader, now have a better hypothesis than they do.

I am glad he mentioned that article, as I had made a note on my iPad: 'Remember to tell him of my relationship with my pill, Temodal, and how I noticed huge mood and energy changes when this summer, with his permission, I stopped taking it in order to be able to play with my son Miro in London.'

I tell him of the sadness I felt as I noticed that, after only four days of being clean from the aggression of that pill, my old body had come back to me and I realized how much I have been missing it. During that little break from my inescapable relationship with a necessary drug, life did look so much better. And now I am back on it, exactly as we had agreed last time. But when I started taking it again, I did feel a real sense of hatred for that little white pill, the one that I swallow every day, and I now know is responsible for sucking my energy away.

After hearing my long-winded tale, Cortesi looked at me carefully and gave me permission to decide by myself, for special occasions, and in particular so I can have the energy to go out and play with Miro, when to stop taking the Temodal.

I don't know what I was expecting to hear from him, but it left me a bit frightened, as my recurring thoughts about not taking that pill, and allowing myself to rely only on my diet and the experimental dendritic vaccine, are only countered by the promise that I give him of taking the pill. He is a scientist and so, even if he likes the work that the vaccine ladies are doing, he has no substantial proof that would allow me to stop my addiction.

I am like an ex-addict who asks his AA mentor if he can go out to a party with a bunch of friends who will surely end up getting drunk. Am I strong enough? Is my relationship with the imaginary future of my son a sufficient excuse?

OK, I'll rely on the fact that, if he says I have to take it, I will do so, and not necessarily because I believe that he and his crew are any better than anyone else (as I have learned, two different top doctors can have a radically different interpretation of my MRIs or blood results), but because he has now become a part of my life, like my neighbourhood in Pigneto in Rome, and like my family in Siena.

When you live through this kind of drama and come out the other side, the relationships are stronger. Not necessarily better, but I've decided to accept them for what they are. Here, I'll show you the man-bag that I sewed for Professor Cortesi.

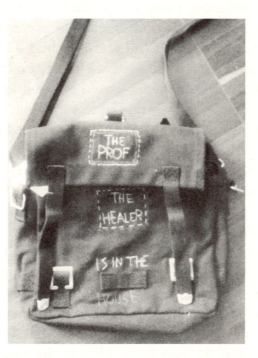

Last time that I was here, Margarita accompanied me, and after the usual positive results she asked the Professor if she could have a private discussion with him, without me. In my absence, she had told him about my insistence on separating (she still does not want to hear the word divorce) and also wanted reassurance that I was healthy enough to take full responsibility for our son, and travel alone with him to London.

She was scared of handing Miro over to me, not so much from an oncological point of view (Cortesi reassured her by saying that if I haven't had any attacks or odd reaction to the pills up to now, I will be fine) but primarily because it would set a precedent that would allow me to travel abroad alone with my son.

That meeting, which was crucial for the further development of our relationship, was possible because both Margarita and I had built trust with him over time, as a human being as well as an oncologist, and that can't be taken for granted. I like Professor Cortesi, because when he has to engage with more complex emotional tensions, he has the capability of switching to an even warmer and more human vocabulary. As well as taking care of my Aliens, he knows that I will always be bouncing issues off him, concerning the changes in my ever more complex personal life.

~

This August I had a truly dreamy vacation playing and running around with Miro without needing to take my two naps a day, and although I often ended up going to sleep a few hours after him, I felt fine. Even the British weather had decided to help us. We went to visit Russell, who was in the countryside finishing off his book about the necessary revolution.

I had organized the trip with Russell's old friend, the comedian Karl Theobald, and his girlfriend, who has a daughter the same age as Miro, and from the very first moment, they got along fantastically. They disappeared in the hills with the two dogs, rode horses, and even managed to encourage each other to swim in the pool without floats.

Russell and I found a calm moment, and he read me a chapter of his book. It is brave and as Russell often manages to be, truly surprising. We talked about his *Happiness* documentary and the new American director who was finally going to complete it. I told him that on the basis of his book, this final turn of events and his change of life, I believe he has managed to create his own ending to that endless *Happiness* documentary. No matter how the director ends up editing the thousand hours of footage that she has in her hands, I know Russell has truly found his own meaning of happiness.

The most precious thing he has is comedy, and he is aware that by taking this even bigger step towards politics with his book, he is at risk of losing it completely. Beppe Grillo, for example, a great Italian comedian who out of desperation entered Italian politics a few years ago, has been taken over by adversarial party games and has totally burned away all of his comedic distance.

But I guess it is exactly the fact that Russell is putting everything he loves at risk that is allowing him to finally find happiness. He has become aware that he will only find peace while contributing to changing the lives of others for the better, and being an active participant in the creation of a fairer life for all; even for those who have nothing. Putting himself and his comedic character in the forefront of a fight, whether it be for human rights or health care, having good schools, having a peaceful place to live, or to be able to give the same status to an immigrant as to your own neighbours, is definitely a tattoo worth getting.

After those few days in the peace of the countryside, Miro and I got back to London, where we explored the beautiful parks and great museums, and occasionally I even took him to a day summer-school to play with proper British kids. One day, coming back from his school in the middle of the council estates by the Barbican Centre, I stopped him on our walk and asked if he needed any new socks or underwear, to which he replied, 'Daddy! These aren't called underwear! Don't you know? These are knickers, Daddy!'

Which brought an almost overwhelming joy to my soul, as all my investment, my stubbornness, those books, films, and invented bedtime stories in English, while he was living in a purely Italian-language world, came back to me. Just eight letters from the mouth of my son, K N I C K E R S (which is probably not even the correct word for a boy's underwear here in London, as I think it is a word only used for girls, but anyway), are proof of the project of which I am proudest to this day: my son speaking English. My boy, already bilingual and embracing the world. If, soon, I am no longer here, that duality of language will continue bouncing around in his brain. Unlike his parents, he is now a native speaker of both English and Italian.

We walked on down the street, while I kept looking at him with his cheeky smile. He was conscious of exactly what he had said and felt almost cocky about his new linguistic superpower. He enjoyed jumping into a school like this and playing and swimming with kids whom he didn't even know, and for that I will always thank his mother, as his social skills are outstanding. I saw him really happy, and so was I.

A few days later:

Miro and I landed back in Rome on a very rainy evening. When we had already entered the door of our house, both soaking wet, Miro jumped back outside with his damp shoes and rang the doorbell continuously for twenty seconds. As I was carrying our suitcases up the stairs, we looked up and saw the faces of Margarita and Jasmina, full of joy. As soon as we walked into the door with our luggage, Margarita kidnapped Miro and took him into the bedroom to kiss him, take off his wet clothes, wash him and listen to all the tales that he urgently wanted to tell her.

I sat in the living room with Jasmina describing our various British experiences, most of which she already knew, as Margarita had made me promise to send her a constant stream of photos, with the whole family copied in. Then Jasmina told me of the apartments they had visited in Trastevere while I was away, and the fact that her opinion still differs radically from her daughter's. On her face, she expressed the most poignant and profound sadness, as if the reality of our separation was overwhelming her.

The apartment that Margarita wants to buy does sound great. I am surprised by how much money they have managed to put together, but that must be, at least in part, from her father Stojan's legacy. As I looked at the floor plan of the house, I told Jasmina how funny it was that it is only 200 metres away from the house where I grew up as a child. That was in the seventies, before gentrification, when that neighbourhood was similar to Pigneto, but now it has become very expensive and probably even more touristy than the Vatican.

Within a few months, before the beginning of the new school year, Margarita and Miro are going to move there to the other side of the city. I discussed this with her before I left for London and from what Jasmina says, she has already started meeting potential renters for our apartment, as I cannot pay for the mortgage and at the same time give her the monthly allowance for Miro that I have promised her.

When Margarita came back into the living room and announced that she was going to get into bed with Miro, I said good night and that we would talk further the next day, while Miro was in school. She looked at me bewildered, raised her arm and pointed towards the door of the house. I had to leave.

While still sitting there in front of Jasmina, I reminded Margarita in my calmest voice, almost pleading, that as I had often done up until then, I could sleep on the couch. If she had a little patience, I would organize my stuff and move to a couch at Blasco's, or Pat and Christina's, tomorrow. Most of my friends knew of our situation and had shown me where to find the sheets and pillows in their houses for those urgent moments.

I remembered that I had a present for Margarita in my suitcase (it was a tradition for me to find something for her in every place I went, and this time I had chosen a particularly nice one, together with Miro), but that evening, there didn't seem to be a way to negotiate anything, not even for one more night.

Margarita is right. I have not been able to take that final

step and physically move out. Take my stuff and go. Leave her to manage her life without me. Why have I been dragging my feet?

Part of it is the fact that I will now need to manage my own life, find ways of dealing with the paperwork of a house, and arrange a financial situation that will allow me to be at home with my boy. But I feel that is only part of it.

I have been nurturing this perception that we might be able to do something radical and reorganize our lives to help each other. You know, be a bit more Scandinavian. Separate houses, separate obligations to each other – but still friends. But you can't do a bit of divorce. Either you commit or it does not make any sense – it only brings pain.

As people who walk into AA groups soon learn, there is no half way. The *only* way is to admit your faults and go 100 per cent clean, and not allow even a little consideration of the fact that you may be strange and ill. In those groups, every single one of them is strange, and also in a deep crisis, and that is not an excuse.

It was now pouring with rain, but I stood up, put on my shoes, and out I went. As the door was closing behind me, I looked at Jasmina, who appeared to be completely overwhelmed and lost.

So here I am . . .

I am outside, waiting for a tram to pass by and take me . . . well, I don't know where. I am getting soaked and my suitcase is getting wetter by the minute. I guess I'll call my friend Blasco, as he's often out in the evening playing with his band of professors and scientists.

Blasco's band has transformed over time (they must have been together for at least twenty years; he was the singer of my band in high school) from punk rock to folk, so I should ask him if they have an old-fashioned country song in their set, which I could use as my soundtrack for this moment. Something very calm and reflective, that can help us follow this story of a lonely man who has left his woman . . . because he is a traveller . . . a gypsy who doesn't know what home is. Or possibly a slightly romanticized version of an idiot, but in any case, it would be great if I could find one of those stray dogs that live around here, who could help me search for a warmer place where I can wait.

OK, it's fine, I'll improvise this part and leave this scene as it is. Having animals on set is always a problem anyway. Yes, he is standing in the rain, holding on his shoulder a bag with all his worldly belongings, watching as all the buses, with their big signs (which even he can read as they are so visual) displaying 'FUORI SERVIZIO' (*Out of Service*), whizz by, splashing dirty water his way. Man, I don't like this kind of production. I have all my nice clothes in this suitcase and I hope at least some of them will stay dry.

Is this the way this story ends? It can't be, as I don't really like being that sad, travelling character. I am tired of me and I am also tired of writing stories about myself, no matter if fictional or real, trying to make sense of my world.

My friend Blasco was really surprised by my call, and seemed angrier with Margarita than me. He told me that he wasn't far away and he would be here in about ten minutes, so I have found a slightly drier place to wait. Right now, I am standing near a big, seventies-built church, where on Sunday the whole neighbourhood meets (or, at least the older citizens of the neighbourhood).

I move to a slightly better place to stand, a bit closer to the church, nearer to the big pine trees, which fortunately haven't been cut down by the work on the new metro station (and God only knows when that will be finished), and are now protecting me from a good part of the rain.

It would be better to tell you this whole story while sitting inside this church. In fact, it is the ideal location to end this book, as the set is perfect, and there is even a fantastic natural background sound of rain bouncing off the windows. I would find a good corner where I could pull off some of my wet clothes . . . and while sitting semi-naked in that church, I could narrate this ending to you. Not bad, right? But I am even wetter, after attempting to open all the different doors, which I guess the priest locks at night to avoid all the drifters and local bums crashing on his narrow wooden benches, so I have to embrace the reality of this ending as it is.

There are many people who survive the horror of their lives by immersing themselves in their computers, but like it or not, at some point a separation – a divorce – does take place. While standing outside this church, I realize the time has also come for me to say goodbye to Alex, and while fondly remembering our endless journeys through this book, the battles with long-winded sentences, struggles with confusing words and annoying repetitions, it is clear even to him that I must put away this computer, away from the rain.

In exactly that moment I am embraced by an infinite calmness. The one that for years Russell had been searching for on his various trips throughout the world. A big smile comes over my face, reminding me of the ending of our production company Vanity Projects and how confident I am that this new beginning is both necessary and healthy.

I have a Finch on the left side of my brain, and no matter what happens along the way, I know that it will help me to fly and transform all my handicaps into new ways of seeing and narrating the comedy and drama of everyday life. It may seem impossible at this moment, but I will attempt to write a new story and read it with my own eyes – with all the artistic benefits of a 'slower' pace of living and the patience that it will require.

The End!

(As I see it, this chapter is exactly ten pages long. ;-))

Appendix

Martino's Five Issues

Lulla Cacioppo
The speech therapist

These are the five issues that prevent Martino Sclavi from being able to read and remember text or to understand its meaning:

1. In the left temporal cerebral regions of the brain, we connect a word with its significance. It analyses the sounds and allows us to recognize their meaning. It makes a mark for each word (like your fingerprints). For Martino, this mark is often not found. It requires quite a lot of patience for him to find, in a manual sense, the meaning. Imagine him as an employee in an old-school office, who compares various fingerprints. He does have those words in his library, but they need to be re-discovered every time.

2. The occipital lobe (amongst many other things) is the visual interpretation that is crucial for reading. There we recognize one meaning of letters, and how one is different from the other. If the ability to recognize these parts is weak or damaged, it is very difficult to identify a word and even harder to access the meaning of a longer sentence.

3. With a deficit in the occipital lobe, like Martino's, there is a reduction of the visual field. Usually, while reading, we are simultaneously looking at a 180-degree spectrum. Considering that Martino's vision is limited, he cannot be aware of what is about to arrive. This hemianopsia gives the effect of a blackout. Over time, patients become aware of this and slowly start moving their head left and right while reading to discover the missing parts.

4. By not being able to see the whole range of text the meanings of words are often confused.

5. Once he finds the correct word, the problem for Martino is to remember its meaning.

All these difficulties do not always appear regularly or simultaneously. They should be considered like a virus in a Word document on the computer, which at times are not active, but at other times are violently blocking all activity.

Acknowledgements

Written words (read back to me from a computer) somehow are not the proper representations of the emotions and the joy necessary for me to thank all the people who saved my life and helped me to turn my battle against text into a truly miraculous friendship. Perhaps I need to do it with a dance or a song . . . or some drawings and kisses . . .

In the absence of such options let me start with a list of people who have saved my life: I have to thank my boy Miro, who constantly reminds me of the importance of loving every minute of life. My crack team of doctors, Margarita Alexievska Sclavi, Prof. Marianella Pirzio Biroli Sclavi and Dr. Bianca Sclavi. I would also like to express my gratitude to Prof. Ada Francia for teaching me how to navigate geographically and psychologically the fields of Roman hospitals. Doctor Marianna Nuti and the whole team working on the dendritic vaccine. Other humans who have definitely saved my life are my oncologist Prof. Cortesi and my surgeon Prof. Santoro in Rome – you both have created space in my head and allowed my finch to dance. Oh, and I definitely have to include Russell Brand among the people who have cut my brain open.

And in no particular order I would also like to express my gratitude to a list of people who have helped me in so many ways: George Lenz and George Milton, who have always kept human relations as the priority of all our pursuits, as well as Nicole Stanner, her mother and, of course, Anna Lenz. Adam Venit for just kicking ass. I must give thanks to Penny Woolcock for lending me her favorite couch to write on, and never allowing me to give up. Jessica Hines, for allowing me to win our bet – you still owe me a cup of tea – and Emily James, for constantly reminding me that the 'impossible' is relative. Lulla Cacioppo for teaching me that understanding reading is not a kid's game. Adrian and the whole Muys family for 27 years of friendship. I have to thank Massimo Sconamiglio for loving art more than his own heart and Valerio Bonelli for reviewing one of my early drafts as if it were a screenplay. Christina Frankopan Nicolson for telling the whole world about my literary endeavours. And thanks to Barry Johnston.

I am particularly indebted to my readers who fed my optimism even when I sent them documents that looked like a complete chaos of misspelled words and only half-conceived chapters. And of course I will make sure to double up on my virtuous dinners for all my friends who have supported my endless couch-surfing endeavours: Susan George, Anna Negri, China Parmalee, Susan Wilk, John Handerson, Tamara Benett-Herrin and Jay Basu, Pat Nicolson, Mark Tilton, Stef Penny and Marco Van Wenzen, Blasco Morozzo and Rossella di Mario, Matteo Morozzo and the entire Morozzo family, Bettina Foa and her dad Vittorio Foa, Martina Meluzzi and the entire Spender family for enlightening my life with wittiness, art and love.

My apologies to all the people whose names I have forgotten – you will always have a place up there in my brain playing around with my finch.

Oh yes, and I have to thank my lovely new entries: my agent Lisa Gallagher and editor Hannah Black.